THE PAIN SOLUTION

The Most Powerful Methods to Heal Yourself

Jack Chapman

Table of Contents

CHAPTER 1

CHAPTER 2

CHAPTER 3

Why You Should Read This Book

Dear Reader,

There is a good chance that if you're reading this book, you either know Jack or you have pain that you need to be gone!

The Pain Solution is the book you need to read and learn about how to get out of pain and stay happy leading a healthy life.

"Jack has acquired some excellent, masterful skills, and knowledge, he imparts it to you in a way that will allow you to understand and apply it immediately in your life."

He is straight to the point and holds you down ensuring you take accountability, and make no excuses for you to take control of your pain and take small steps to take action immediately.

The knowledge in this book has the power to help and inspire you to create a pain-free lifestyle. When followed regularly coupled with exercises, Jack gives his clients and himself and uses them every day to empower both confidence and creativity for a healthy life balance.

This book is a self-help guide with many tips and exercises that have been helpful to many of my clients. Each person is different but some of these ideas will work for most.

No One Got Better by Not Taking Action!

Disclaimer

—•◦∞◦•—

Neither the author nor the publisher will guarantee that anyone following any of these techniques, ideas, and exercises will get out of pain or become pain-free due to medical conditions or medication currently being undertaken.

The author and publisher shall have neither liability nor responsibility to anyone with respect to any loss, illness, or damage caused or alleged to be caused, directly or indirectly by the information contained in this book.

If you are unsure about your health, please seek advice from your GP or Health Practitioner.

ISBN: 9798379189594

Copyright - Jack Chapman ACMT 2023

Foreword

—————•◯◯•—————

Dear Reader,

It is with great pleasure that I write this foreword for this book, which delves into self help for chronic pain in an accessible and thoughtful way. This book is a culmination of extensive clinical practice with real people, deep insights and practical wisdom, offering a comprehensive understanding of the subject.

Jack has done an excellent job of presenting the material in a clear and concise manner, making it accessible to all. The case studies, and practical exercises provide a hands-on approach to learning, making it easy for you, the reader, to grasp and apply the concepts discussed.

This book is not just limited to providing knowledge, but also offers practical solutions to the challenges faced in dealing with chronic pain issues. Jack has expertly blended theoretical knowledge with practical insights, making it a valuable resource for anyone looking to deepen their understanding of how to help themselves out of pain

It is my hope that this book will inspire you to think critically, challenge your existing beliefs, and provide you with the tools and knowledge to make a difference in your own life and in the lives of others.

Thank you for choosing to read this book and I hope you find it as enlightening and informative as I did.

Sincerely,

Rachel Fairweather

Director Jing Institute of Advanced Massage
BA, Dip SW, CQSW, AOS Massage Therapy

Testimonials for - The Pain Solution

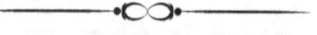

"This is simply Jack at his best!

"His compassionate understanding of both people and the body is shared in this book that provides practical solutions to create a positive change. I'm in!"

Lois Norman – UK

Performance and Life Coach

www.loisnorman.org

"Jack is very focused & determined with his studies which makes him an expert in his field. He has surprised and inspired me in a number of ways over the years, he is very motivated and shows so much care to all his friends and clients."

Mandy Rawsthorne - Kent UK

Author of - Now Is Your Time

www.fit2relax.org

"This book addresses some valuable issues related to the rehabilitation of aches, pains, and injuries and provides cutting-edge information regarding tissue injury and repair.

Not only does optimal rehabilitation assist in returning an injured person to training but a carefully administered programme serves to prevent the reoccurrence of the same injury or the occurrence of additional injuries.

Thus, the main objective of Jack's work is to provide an easily digested overview of the principles of sports rehabilitation. Many people suffer needlessly from pain and discomfort and much of this can be relieved quickly and effectively from reading his work."

Kimberley-Ann Jones

Ms Olympia Competitor

Master Gym Trainer

London UK

www.keepitmoving.co.uk

What My Clients Are Saying About Me

—————•◯◯•—————

I was on a course and unfortunately, I hurt my back. Luckily for me Jack was on the course and he offered to help me out, after about 15 minutes of working on my back it felt so much better! I then had a 2-hour drive home and there is no way I would have been able to do it without Jack's help! I wish I lived closer to Jack as I would go to him again! I can highly recommend him :-) Thanks again, Jack!

- Natasha-

Professional, knowledgeable, and friendly to name a few of Jack's qualities. I have been Jack's client for a few years now and he has always been the only one able to put me back on track, even while dealing with pregnancy's usual pain. His consultation at the beginning of every appointment is detailed and focused on the individual requirement and so are the treatment and recommended exercises he provides. His client's safety and well-being are his drive. I highly recommend him.

– Angela-

I cannot recommend Jack enough, to the point where I have now recommended him to friends and family who are now also regulars. He got recommended to me by my partner who has seen him for years and first found him on Google. He is very experienced and comes with a vast amount of knowledge. He takes his time to not only ask about you to get to know you but also gives you stretches to go away and practice. He provides a good assessment by looking at your range of movement when you first arrive as well as looking into your pain areas. He then explained the different types of headaches I was getting and why, along with explaining what trigger points are and what techniques he will be using. He has worked wonders on my shoulder blades, neck muscles, back muscles, tight hamstrings, and calves which have resulted in my migraines stopping. He has a lovely space for his treatments, which is a very calming area, beautifully decorated, always clean, and, very well organized and equipped. I now continue to see Jack regularly for monthly maintenance sessions and only wish I found him earlier. He is a man of many talents and does a lot of other avenues of work, including supporting his community and providing exercise classes, particularly for stroke patients. Thank you.

- Nat-

Jack is definitely the go-to therapist. Along with general massage, he does specific area treatments using unique clinical techniques. He's very thorough, knowledgeable, and happy to impart information. After being attended to by various other professionals who either couldn't find or couldn't treat me, I had an awesome treatment with Jack, who readily found and spent over an hour treating it in one hit. He gave good aftercare advice and exercises. Highly recommend.

– Pamela-

I couldn't even bend over to do up my shoes, you are very reassuring and I felt comfortable that you knew exactly what my issue was

- Caroline-

Had pain today in my shoulder and went to see Jack Chapman after a Google search. He was able to see me on the same day. Had one treatment and could see the difference straight away. Highly recommend Jack. Many thanks Jack for today and see you at the next time.

- Jaspal-

Having suffered from chronic neck & shoulder pain after a car accident many years ago I tried numerous therapies that did not work. Then I found Jack, he is absolutely amazing, he has done complete wonders. Very talented individual. Highly recommend!

– Kate-

I see Jack for help with maintaining my pain levels associated with severe Fibromyalgia and Arthritis. Each treatment is tailored to my needs on the day. Treatment for me has included various types of massage, manipulation and stretches. Jack is very well informed and a highly qualified clinical massage therapist. He assesses, treats and also offers advice to avoid reaching a crisis point. He suggests specific strengthening exercises and stretches. He has a private, dedicated space for treatment which is clean and calming. My conditions result in pain, discomfort, stiffness, and chronic fatigue. Visiting Jack keeps me mobile and able to continue a reasonably independent lifestyle. Jack is friendly and very professional and I do not hesitate in recommending him.

– Sonia-

I regularly have a massage for my weak shoulder and back and always feel much better afterwards. I would highly recommend booking an appointment with Jack Chapman as the service provided is very professional and the therapist is extremely qualified in his profession.

– Lea-

Acknowledgements

—•◯◯•—

Firstly, I would like to thank my family and friends who have supported and believed in me on my long journey to be the best version of myself to help and inspire others.

I'd also like to thank the various teachers and mentors that have changed me, and made me stronger and wiser in some shape or form, your inspiration is incredible and will always travel with me.

I've had the privilege to cross paths with strong individuals and learn from both Rachel Fairweather and Meghan S Mari two of the most compassionate and wise bodyworkers I've ever known. Business coaches have never stopped pushing me and checking in. Rita Nash for the big dreams I once had, I can now drive anywhere around the world.

To my long-term friend from back in the day when the gym was the real deal Kimberley-Ann Jones for your professional drive. Charlie Kiss who left us too soon, a true brave influencer and follower of his dreams, and to Lea Flower for your strength and courage dear cousin to just get it done, do it and carry on against all odds, we survive under oppression.

To many others that I've not mentioned here at this moment you know who you are.

I'd just like to say again

Thank you

A TEACHER - Takes A Hand, Opens The Mind, And Touches The Heart

To my little cat Magic, who I often see from my living room window waiting for me, welcoming me back on my returns from clients and days away while working and training to help others - thank you for your loving companionship little one.

Thank you Nan for your huge influence and guidance in my early years and your guidance today. You knew more about me than I knew myself back then.

I wish I'd known what I know now and helped you with your pain at times thereby giving back to you. Sometimes I can still see you and hear your wise voice and it brings a sad smile.

Dedication

——————•⃝∞⃝•——————

This book is dedicated to all the body workers around the world that help so many, your touch and compassion is priceless

CHAPTER
1

The Pain Solution

It's all in your head Mrs Jones

How often have you heard the phrase "It's all in your mind" or "You're making it all up Mrs Jones"? This is sometimes the case with clients at their GP Surgery especially with clients suffering from pain conditions such as Arthritis or Fibromyalgia which are part of the Arthritis family that comes and goes with stress, diet and inflammation which can make it all much worse in the long run.

Definition of pain

A localized or generalized unpleasant bodily sensation or complex of sensations that causes mild to severe physical discomfort and emotional distress and typical results from bodily disorder such as injury or disease.

Why do we get pain?

Pain is felt as protection meconium to protect the body when we have damaged or hurt ourselves. It alerts us of the danger and acts as a warning for us not to carry on and to stop whatever will be doing.

Pain types

There are different types of pains and here is the list below:

- Nerve Pain – Touches nerves i.e., Sciatic, Spinal cord

- Chronic Pain – Nagging ongoing over time from conditions

- Stabbing /Sharp Pain – Paper Cut, Trip, Twisting, New Injury

We get pain in different ways

- ### In the short term

  Pain can happen at any time be it a trip, slip, reaching or a twist and immediate pain followed by a thought of, Am I ok?, Can I move?, What have I done?, Can I get up?, Who saw me?, sod that bloody thing i.e., Short term pain is normally so quick we jump to defend ourselves and pass the blame onto humiliation or frustration.

- ### Long time coming

  This could be a build-up of pain over time due to workload, stress, posture, not taking breaks, working long hours or not dealing with the pain when it first started a while back, years in fact. Long-time pain is normally slow and our own doing i.e. – we could have done something to have avoided it.

- ### YoYo Of pain

  Picture this: you have a lower back pain due to over working, you go to the GP they give you painkillers and refer you for physio, you stop working so much and do your exercises, and your back pain stops over a short time. So, you get back to your workload as your back pain is better, and then you forget to exercise (no time you're busy working). Guess what? Back pain comes back and round we go again.

It's a bit like dieting, gaining and losing weight up down up down so would it not be wiser to maintain the exercises and work smarter so as not to cause the reaction above?

What do we mean? Finding ways to stop pain from occurring.

Years ago, I would do five massages a day and, by the end of the week I would be tired and my back ached. I saw a chiropractor; I didn't exercise enough and slowly I was burning out.

Then came Covid and work ethics changed thanks to Zoom, and so did my work, for the better. I set up stretch sessions three times a week for clients. I also took up running once a week and ended up losing, 3 plus stone in weight. I did less massage work in person and more teaching in Rehab and On–Line, as clients were getting better, so was I.

Something to think about

- **Office worker**

  Try to do the following: Fix your office desk and chair, computer height, take lunch breaks, drink water, eat nutritious food , sleep 8 hours, try not to sit for long, stretch, exercise, walk, and swim before or after work etc.

  Don't sit for hours and hours without a break. It might not be easy as you get caught up in computer work, but since Covid, many people people now work from home, so there's no excuse for not taking a break. A great one is to take a walk at lunchtime and get out in the fresh air.

- **Builder**

  Taking breaks, lunch breaks, 8 hours of sleep, drinking water, nutrition, gym, walking before or after work, varying work will avoid RSI on hand, wrist and forearms or being on knees, crouching under sinks also takes its toll on your lower back.

  I hear this a lot from builders "My job is so physical I don't need to exercise", Ok but being physical is not exercise or stretching, it's very different.

  What do you eat for lunch? – Café fry ups? Ok, why don't you try taking a packed lunch, making a protein drink with some fruit or choosing something healthier.

- **A note**

  Just because a family member has for instance,. arthritic knees or lumbar pain doesn't mean you will have too , don't let that be your final answer. It's all too easy to blame or say "It's genetic or because my Mum had xxx, I will too". Think about your lifestyle and what you can do to change to avoid this. What didn't they do that I can do?

There are four types of people with different characters

There're four types of people with different characters, when it comes to Getting out Of Pain

1. **"Let's work together Client"**

   This client will do whatever it costs and whatever they need to do to "Get out Of Pain"- This is the therapists' ideal client.

2. **"The Coper"**

   This client works well with their therapist in getting the healing process underway. They will stick to your goals and vision.

3. **"Fix Me Now Client"**

   This client expects a miracle cure but they don't want to help themselves in any way by doing the stretching and homework that's set. Often with excuses such as: " I forgot to" and rush to get back to exercise and sports too soon.

4. **"The Avoider"**

   This client works closely with the 'Fix Me Client' to avoid things at all costs and 'bury your head in the sand', hoping it will all go away.

Why we hold on to pain for so long

Talking to clients during consultations, it's not unusual for them to hold on to pain for several years. I used to find this quite alarming and thought people would like the pain to go as quickly as it came , until I started to realise a number of things with people.

Subconsciously this is what is going on in our minds when it comes to pain:

1. Pain becomes a talking point for me

2. I am playing the victim with my pain

3. I am not ready to let go of my pain yet

4. My pain reminds me of a past incident, trauma or an unpleasant event

5. Pain can become my trophy or a battle wound card

6. It becomes part of my everyday life and it becomes the norm over time

7. I don't know what to do to get rid of my pain

8. Who can help me get rid of my pain?

9. I don't take action due to a lack of funds

10. I am too busy to find the time or a therapist to sort it out

11. I am hoping it will all go away

12. It will never work for me, my family had the same condition

EXERCISE

What number between 1 – 12 above, best describes your current situation?

My current situation is best described as Number

....

Why do you think it's this number?

....
....

Remember

1. It's never too late to do something to help yourself with pain.

2. The longer it's left the more its memory leaves a blueprint on the body.

I Can't (at the moment)

How to Help Yourself

- Take personal responsibility for your pain.

Ever had a friend with pain and you ask them:

How are you?

- **Friend 1**

  "A little back pain but nothing to stop me from working with it and then going shopping in the evening, getting on with it".

  They're not interested in a reply or a sympathy vote from anyone – i.e., The Copier. (They have a positive mindset, they're working, socializing and moving around getting on with life.)

  This person will go on to becoming injury and pain free in a short space of time.

- **Friend 2**

  "Arh, my back pain I am in agony, I lay in bed all day yesterday tossing and turning, I took four painkillers and posted to the world about it all over Facebook."

  They look at you waiting for a response to say – poor you i.e. The Avoider (They have a hindered mindset, they're staying at home, off work, not moving, and are looking for a sympathy vote i.e. – Playing the Victim) This person will take a longer time to become pain and injury free.

  The Coper and the Let's Work Together Client. On this one, the therapist has a job getting this client out of pain and getting a good result for the client. Overall therapists love referrals and a good reputation.

  The Avoider and the Fix Me Now Client. We know you are not helping yourself and only come to see us when you're in pain and don't do your stretches. You also do not take our advice nor put it into practice regularly. We know who you are and we will do our best to help you though we are not expecting great results. If we can fit you in, we will but a home truth, really, you're just wasting your money and our time.

The Avoider	The Coper
Worries too much	Does not worry
Gets frightened by the pain	Knows that the pain will pass
Rests too much	Carries on without moaning
Afraid of damaging themselves	Gets on with life
Waits for the pain to go away	Does Exercises & Stretching
Withdraws from life	Stays active and positive

Avoiders	Copers
Have pain for longer than it needs to be	Pain goes away fast and quick
Time off from work, Sickness	Stays as active and healthy
Can become disabled over time	Gets over the Pain & moves on

The Fix Me Now Client	Lets work together Client
Doesn't take responsibility for their Pain	Takes Responsibility for their Pain
I've been too busy to ice my knee but I played football over the weekend	
No I forgot to do any exercise you told me	Yes I've iced my knee twice a day
Too Busy to fit time in for appointments	Yes I've been to yoga and swimming Makes Regular Appointments
One Session will fix me again	I'll book today for 6 x sessions
It is really two years since my last session	I'll book again next week right now
I'd rather spend my money on a bigger car	My health is important to me
No Sorry I haven't been drinking much water	Yes I've doubled my water intake
I haven't stretched at all this week	Stretching really helped this week

Let's take the results from the Avoider & Fix Me, Client

I am still in pain it must be the therapist's fault, not mine. It's not my problem I am still in pain.

Stupid therapist, fancy asking me to book 6 sessions and do all those silly stretches, ice, and heat. That is what I pay them to do. FIX ME, I am too busy, they're only out to make money and I am still in pain.

DIFFERENT ATTITUDE – DIFFERENT OUTCOME

Let's take the results from the Coper & Let's Work Together Client

I am getting so much better, I can see the results now over the past couple of sessions and I feel great, I am glad I spent the time and money looking after my health.

The Therapist is really understanding and the stretches and tips he has given are really helping, I am almost pain free.

What can you do right now to help yourself? It all starts with you

EXERCISE

Be honest with yourself there are no right or wrong answers you will just be clearer about helping yourself in the future.

1. **What category do you think you fall into?**

   A. The Avoider

   B. Fix Me Now

   C. The Coper

   D. Lets Work Together

2. **What do you think is the biggest thing holding you back from getting Out of Pain?**

   A. ....

   B. ....

   C. ....

   D. ....

3. **What two things could you do right now to help yourself with your pain?**

(i.e. – Do some stretching, get an extra hour's sleep tonight, drink water etc

1. ....

2. ....

Go and get your diary and mobile phone

Google - Jing Massage Brighton – www.jingmassage.com

(Jing Massage Therapists are the UK's highest trained Massage Therapists in the UK)

Look up your nearest Jing Clinical Massage Therapist and book a couple of sessions with them.

Start helping yourself NOW!

Reflective Questions

What was the most valuable message you received in this chapter?

The most valuable message I received in this chapter was: ....
....
....
....
....

Which Two things from this Chapter will you try to help reduce your pain?

1. ....
....
....
....

2. ....
....
....
....

What will you do differently from now on?

I will

....
....
....
....
....
....
....
....
....

NOTES

CHAPTER 2

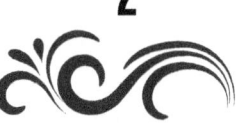

Pain Killers (Behind The Mask)

If I had a pound for every client that had been to their GP and was only given pain killers or an injection and told to rest and that it will all be fine, I'd be retired by now.

Some GP's advice goes something like this –

GP – "How can I help you?"

You – I've hurt my xxxx

GP – "Mr Smith you will need to

Rest, stop the activity, here's a prescription for – XXX

If you're overweight – Then eat and exercise better

Do You Smoke? - Then stop smoking.

GP- If it's no better in a week come back and see me

You OK thank you

Most people don't bother to go back as the waiting time for appointments is too long nowadays and it's not a GP's main remit to know how to deal with pain conditions. They're hoping that the above prescription will sort it out for a while.

They haven't got time to go through your history about how you got your pain and God help you if you have more than one painful area as nowadays you can only ask them to help with one thing at a time.

If you do go back, you may be sent off for various tests which include:

- ✓ Blood tests
- ✓ Urine Sample
- ✓ Hydrotherapy
- ✓ Bone Density Scan
- ✓ MRI Scan, X–Ray, CT Scan
- ✓ Ultra Sound / Tens Therapy
- ✓ Physio (given a sheet of exercises)

Pain killers

There are so many types of pain killer drugs. You might be familiar with some of these:

- ✓ Co-Codamol
- ✓ Ibuprofen
- ✓ Diclofenac
- ✓ Naproxen
- ✓ Tramadol
- ✓ Gabapentin
- ✓ Diazepam
- ✓ Morphine

Each painkiller is given for the role it plays in reducing inflammation, lifting moods and how it affects the central nervous system. These pain killers come in various formats such as liquid, tablets and patches, all of which can help manage your pain.

Many people will start taking the prescription and find horrible side effects that affect them. This may result in them stopping taking them and finding themselves not better off than when they started them.

Common Side Effects – Constipation, Nausea (sickness) Drowsiness, etc.

What the prescription would have done is mask the pain and given the pain condition time to settle for a while.

The GP would not have time to answer your biggest questions or get to the root cause. This is because you can't take a pain consultation in 5 minutes and they are also too busy dealing with too many people in the NHS System so you are just a number.

So now what?

X-Ray, MRI & CT scans

What does it all mean?

Most people have gone for one of these or have heard of them, but what do they do and what do they help you in finding out?

X – Ray – Electromagnetic X – Radiation

Looking at bones and joints for fractures and bone breaks.

- **MRI Scan – Magnetic Resonance Imaging**

  They use magnetic fields and radio waves to generate images of the organs in the body. It involves you lying inside a tube during the scan

- **CT scan - Computed Tomography Scan**

  CT Scan computer processes combinations for bone disorders, fractures, blood clots and diseases.

- **Ultra Sound – Sometimes called a Sonogram**

Uses high frequency sound waves that create an image of the inside of the body's soft tissue defects or blockages.

- **TENS Machine – TENS Transcutaneous**

  Battery-powered device that uses electrodes to stimulate nerves on the skin to help block or suppress pain.

What have you tried so far?

Most people I have spoken to have tried some form of therapy or sought help from elsewhere and the question remains, did they work?

The Choice is huge where do you start?

1. Relaxation Massage

If you're lucky you may find a nice, polite young lady in a nylon tunic who only went to Massage School for a weekend to a month course, but she's quite good and can give you a relaxation massage that makes you feel relaxed and gets rid of a couple of knots. Usually, fundamental information is taken while the whale music plays and the waft of lavender oils will be filling the air. After finishing, she says, "I'll leave you here for a few minutes to redress, you come out when you have finished" and when you do, you will never see her again. She would have already moved on to her next client so there's no feedback for you.

2. Chiropractor

With a full-size skeleton friend called Skelly in the corner of the room. After having your neck and arms pulled across your body to adjust your spine and be cracked in various positions and be tapped with high power hammer tools that feel like an electric staple gun (without the staples) while still dressed then be asked to get up and walk around he ushers you out and on to his next client in a rushed 15 minutes flat.

3. Physio

Usually set in a Medical White Clinical Room with a straight to the point stern attitude, they ask you to "turn this way, that foot needs to be here, you're not leaning far enough."

20 Minutes later after adjusting your body to its exact millimetre position and 6 Free NHS sessions of this if you're lucky and their job is done, whether you're still in pain or not, back on the NHS LONG waiting list if you need more.

A programme called Physio Tools that has a few picture exercises for you to do and chances are no one follows them as they're not shown what to do or there is no one to encourage them to perform them daily.

4. Sports Massage

Not for the faint hearted but most people think it's just what they need, more pain. Like it or not this is my pressure No Pain No Gain is their motto like it or not as you squirm your face into the face cradle and silent tears roll down your face. I'll fix you in one session with my foam roller and iron bar up your calf then wrap you with Sports Tape that will give you a free wax. Leaving you in dire agony or bruised to a pulp to limp out of the sports room to recover with more pain than you came in with. Would you dare to go back for the next bash-in?

5. Reflexology

Most people want to try this as a last resort, laying back on a garden chair recliner fully dressed with your trouser legs rolled up while the Reflexologist sprays and wipes your feet then proceeds to press and pull your feet and circle your toes then repeat on the other foot.

The Reflexologist then finishes by pressing kidney one in the ball of your foot to relax you, chances are it was relaxing and you will sleep well tonight.

6. Acupuncture

If you're a stick for needles you'll love this one. Like a human pin cushion with very fine needles with fancy spindle wire that if you're lucky may set light to the end, let you smoulder while another needle is inserted into your skin.

Acupuncture isn't as bad as it sounds and doesn't hurt half as much as you think.

7. Yoga

Someone told you you need gentle stretching or flexibility, right? Seek your yoginis out in a local church hall or yoga centre for this one. Lovely to relax and fantastic for your mind and flexibility but be aware that you may end up with your ankle around your neck called the Pig Pose-Om.

8. Local Gym

Lycra lovers and mirror hogs on their mobile phones, pumping out the big weights, much more than they can really handle with bad form and too much distraction. If you have been to the gym don't go in peak time, you'll never get a machine or a pair of dumbbells to match. It will be too busy and full of Cardio Electric runners on their mobiles, posing in front of the mirror's thinking they're Arnold.

9. Liquid Pain Killers (Gold Injections, Cortisone Shots)

Inflammation-blocking agents used for joint pain, arthritis, and tendonitis, used to dampen the pain, take 3-5 days to work and can last for a couple of weeks. They are usually injected into the Buttock or joint area and given for Frozen Shoulder pain conditions called Adhesive Capsulitis. They still come with the side effects much the same as Pain Killers

10. Nothing

Nothing will get better than doing nothing.

So there you have it take your pick and try them out one may just work for you!!!

Exercise

Which one will you try?

....

....

....

....

....

Using Ice and Heat

Ice

Ice helps slow blood flow to an injury, reducing inflammation, swelling and pain. It should be used right away after an injury. It also is excellent for - sprains, strains, bumps, slips, trips, falls, burns and headaches. Here is how ice works:

- Ice in the first 24 – 48 hours of injury.

- A packet of frozen peas in a pillowcase, cover works and moulds around a limb well as an Ice pack to stop painful spasms and inflammation.

- Don't put ice directly on your skin and leave it, it can cause an ice burn just like a heat burn.

- 15 minutes at a time, then wait an hour in between.

- An iced bottle can be good for rolling on your foot for Planter injuries.

If you are ever in doubt if it's ice or heat to use – use ice.

Heat

Heat is great to loosen up stiff joints and tight muscles. It opens up blood vessels which increase blood flow and help to alleviate pain. Heat should be used 72 hours after an injury. Heat is great for – loosening up stiff, tight muscles and chronic pain. Here is how heat works:

- A hot water bottle in a pillow case cover works well as a heat pack.

- A radiator or silver towel rail works well to stand against your clothes, just be careful they get hot.

- Don't fall asleep with the heat on an area as you may burn yourself if left on too long.

Spiky & Hard Ball

Most people will have a hard ball around the house, be it a dog ball, tennis ball, golf ball or spiky ball from the laundry. This is one tool that will do wonders if used in the right way and can offer fast relief for pain.

Ball Foot Rolling

Place the ball under the sole of your naked foot while standing and roll away, not too fast you need to roll the ball very mindfully, you're looking for any soft or tender areas, in particular the, bridge back to the heel and under your toes. At first attempt, it will probably be a little unpleasant, but as time goes on the more you do it the easier it will become, and the pain will lessen.

Exercise

Bend over and slowly see how far you can touch your toes; just monitor how far you can go and how tight your hamstrings at the upper back legs feel.

Now do the ball rolling as above, spending three minutes or so on each foot. Now try again to bend over and touch your toes, this time it should be a lot easier and the hamstrings in your back legs should be not so tight.

What you have done is to open up some of your artificial back line that runs from head to foot.

Other uses

A hard ball or spikey ball can also be used as a mini foam roller to work on the soles of your feet, hips, glutes and lumber, any tight areas that you can find while leaning against a wall and slowly working around the tight area.

A sponge or soft ball on the other hand is better for people with arthritis and gaining hand strength due to hand injuries and also great for stroke clients gaining hand grip.

A golf ball in a long sock over the shoulder leaning against a wall can do wonders for self-treating shoulder and shoulder blade areas. The long sock prevents the ball from dropping on the floor each time you move or roll.

Knowledge is Power

One thing I've learnt is, no matter how many tries, some people still don't listen or take your advice, and as a therapist, you can only help to a certain level but you still have to help yourself and YES do your homework.

A therapist is like a friendly school teacher

Remember therapists see results in clinics all the time and know that some things work better than others although it isn't the same for everyone, each person and treatment is different.

Therapists have heard all the excuses under the sun. Excuses like:

I didn't get time, I am not a morning person, I don't like exercise, and I don't like drinking plain water.

I worked in gyms in my teens and have heard all the excuses under the sun not to exercise or to get out of a situation.

Once you get into a routine or habit keep it going, if you fall out of the routine start it again as soon as possible or you will end up falling off the wagon and stopping.

Start with one or two new things a week, otherwise, it can get overwhelming.

Back in the early 90's when I was doing heavy training for Bodybuilding competitions and working full-time in gyms. I would see an increase in people between January (New Year) and July (Holidays). This routine with keen newbies continues to this day and I often laugh with my PT gym instructor friends about this even now.

Why come January, do you think new gym members stop 8 weeks down the line?

YES, they're all eager to start their new diet or exercise programme but have done too much too quickly and have stopped due to lifting too heavy, going too often or new pain and the enthusiasm doesn't last.

Questions asked can be –

Did you xxxxxxx? STRETCH

Did you use xxxxxx? YOUR BALL/ BAND

Did you get enough xxxxxxx? SLEEP

Did you eat xxxxxxx? ENOUGH PROTEIN

Did you try not doing xxxxxxx? THAT FOOTBALL OR RUN

Did you drink more   xxxxxxxx? WATER

Stay on track

EXERCISE

Grab a pen and paper and mark out Monday to Sunday and work out a time that's good for you to do your exercises

For example:

Monday	Tuesday	Wednesday	Thursday	Friday	Saturday	Sunday
Gym				Walk		
	Stretch		Stretch		Stretch	

Now get your diary and write on what days you are planning to go to the gym or do your exercises etc.

Now get your mobile and set a reminder and set up an app to remind you to drink water

(It may be when you get up, it may be lunchtime, it may be later in the evening while settling down.)

*Wake up, do your stretches while lying on the bed, pop to the bathroom grab a glass of water on the way back to the bedroom, you've achieved two actions already - stretching and drinking more water.

*10 minutes or 1 - 2 stretches is better than doing nothing.

*Have a goal in mind and have a mindset that you are doing the necessary actions to reach your goal.

*Clothes ironed hanging on a rail, shoes polished and bag packed - saves time

*A mug with a teabag, spoon, and the kettle full and ready to boil - saves time

*A packed lunch with a bottle of water all ready to take out from the fridge - saves time

In a minute

One minute is all it takes to do 1 x stretch that helps maintain your flexibility and movement and the all-important - Keeping you out of pain

But I hear all the time from clients –

"I don't have enough time"

"I am too busy"

Really, your pain can't be that bad then ….

So here is a list of 12 ideal times to be able to stretch, so now you have no excuse …

Don't worry about what you look like just get on and do them.

1. Sitting on the bus or train = everyone is too busy on their phone to even notice you.

2. Waiting at traffic lights while driving = some lights take forever to

change.

3. Waiting for the kettle to boil for a brew = At least 2 - 3 x minutes.

4. Sitting on the loo, people read = Why can't you stretch?

5. While watching TV = during the all-important adverts.

6. While you're waiting for the microwave to ping = while heating something.

7. While travelling up an escalator or in a lift = with a big mirror to monitor progress.

8. In a queue, on your phone with the hold music or waiting to be served at a till.

9. Set your alarm 10 minutes earlier in the morning or just before you go to sleep.

10. On your lunchtime break, I have lots of time to stretch or go for a relaxing walk.

11. While in the cinema, during the coming soon trailers = No one can see you in the dark.

12. While you're waiting between courses at a restaurant table = There's lots of time,

Plan ahead

Get up earlier

Structure your week

Get a diary, a calendar or a mobile scheduler. –We all should know the hospital, dentist, massage appointments, birthdays, and bin day. But do you know when you're going to call X, when the dog's vaccination is due, when the car needs to go for its MOT, and what day you are going out for dinner?

Make a plan

If you're working get into a routine, you know your working hours, and rest days

If you're Self Employed ask yourself – I run this business what hours do I wish to work, rest and play?

What days am I on holiday this year, when are the kids on holiday, when is the gas bill due to go up?

What day in the week is – food shopping day, hair cut day, clothes washing day, social going out day, gardening day, tidying / cleaning day, washing and hovering the car/ can day etc.?

Get busy the night before

I don't care what time you finished work make sure these things get done tonight. It will make the morning so much simpler.

Set your alarm so that you are not late again, get your clothes/uniform and shoes polished ready and hung up. Get your packed lunch ready to go in the fridge. Fill the kettle with water, get a cup and spoon ready with a tea bag at least you get a cup before you leave for work. Take note, breakfast is a must.

In the evenings

Get out and go for a walk 2 - 3 times a week. Take the dog, he'll love you for it as well and it will allow you to unwind and create some quiet time to think. If you 've been stuck in an office all day or on a building site stuck on your knees, under a sink don't just plonk down and watch Corrie.

(I once had a client sleep for 8 hours a day, sat at a desk all day working, then sat all evening watching TV no exercise at all and wondered why he was in so much pain and his lower back & knees hurt him)

Stretch – You know you should be stretching and you'll feel so much better for it, try aiming for 4/5 times a week if in pain or twice a week just for maintenance to keep you mobile.

Stop a moment

Ever had that feeling when you have so many things to do that it's overwhelming?

Stop and think about what things need doing now? Is it life or death?

Can I get someone else to do this or help me?

What things can wait until later or tomorrow?

Make a list so you don't forget what you needed to do.

What things am I doing just for the sake of doing something?

Don't waste time we can never get it back once it's gone.

Busy being busy, doing what exactly, what are you doing?

Procrastination

We can all procrastinate; procrastination is the thief of time, and when we don't want to do something, we put it off. It suddenly becomes very important to check our mobile phones, email and ev en though you hate housework it becomes important to push the hover around.

Anything to avoid the main task of exercise or stretching because it's not a habit or in your daily routine. As I've said before if you get into a habit or routine your life becomes easier and simpler.

Rewards

It does wonders to reward yourself for a task or job well done. It keeps you motivated and moving forward especially working or living alone, to recognize and acknowledge yourself; nothing lavish unless you want to, but a bunch of flowers is just the ticket.

Six Doctors of Health

(Most of these we can do daily and are even free and require little time)

Fresh Air - Nature, Breathe, Stress

Sunshine – Mood, Happy, Vitamin D, Health

Rest – Recover, Repair, Growth, Stress

Food – Nutrition, Repair, Growth, Health

Water – Energy, Pain, Hydration

Exercise – Health, Weight, Pain, Stress

Reflective Questions

What was the most valuable message you received in this chapter?

The most valuable message I received in this chapter was

....
....
....
....
....
....

Which two things from this chapter will you try to help your pain?

1 ---

2 ---

What will you do differently from now on?

NOTES

If You Put Your Mind To It, You Can Do Anything To Want To You Just Have To Believe And Take Action

1-2-3 Let's Go .....

CHAPTER
3

Nan's Neck

Years ago, when I was in my teens, my grandmother had arthritis in her neck and spine. She was told to wear a high braced white plastic neck collar when the arthritis was bad, and to keep her neck still.

She was not given any exercises to do, to help with flexion or rotation so lived off painkillers when it was very bad.

Do you see people with neck collars nowadays for arthritis – No?

New ways of thinking and research have changed this, somehow, I wish she was around now. I could have helped her so much with the knowledge I now have.

Attitude

People's attitude to pain is still based on the old school way of thinking, how often when someone has a painful back do you hear -

I need to lay down on a hard floor

I need to go and lay in bed all day

NO

You should be moving, walking around and stretching it out in a safe and steady way.

Even First Aid has changed –

RICE – Rest, Ice, Compression, Elevation

MICE – Movement, Ice, Compression, Elevation

Nothing changes if nothing changes

(I love this quote)

Think about this for a minute....

Nothing changes

So nothing will change, it will stay the same if you do nothing

If nothing changes

If you don't change something or do something different

** YOU are the one to do this –It starts with YOU

No one is going to do it for you, you need to do it for YOU and if you really want it you will do it and if you don't well then you'll make all the excuses under the sun.

Rehabilitation Is Hard Enough, Now It's Up To You. Will You Still Be In The Same Place If I Visited You A Year From Now?

Reflective Questions

What was the most valuable message you received in this chapter?

The most valuable message I received in this chapter was:

Which two things from this chapter will you try to help your pain?

1. --

What will you do differently from now on?

NOTES

Why Is My Progress So Slow And Why Am I Not Getting Any Better?

CHAPTER
4

We are Detectives

During a consultation, people forget about their habits and home behaviours and it can be like playing detective for us therapists, asking questions and listening to pick up clues and signs along the way until you end up with an image in your head linking the puzzle pieces together.

A great massage therapist will ask you lots of questions. We're interested to know how you are moving and how much exercise you're getting.

Years of working as a real live store detective and then in the Security Department at a high-profile London Embassy, checking bodies, bags, cars, and posts for explosives has helped me be a good detective, seeking out information and adding the puzzle pieces together.

With one client it turned out that he got up in the morning at 7.00am after lying in bed for 8 hours, then sat all day in his home office from 8.00. am to 6.00pm, then spent all evening watching television from 7.00pm until 10.30pm until he went to bed again at 11.00pm. We added in some exercise and he now walks his dog at lunchtime and in the evening and plays golf on the weekend.

We are interested to know the water you're drinking for recovery and hydration purposes.

A client once told me that all they drink in a day was three cups of tea, it was only a third of his daily intake, 1 litre.

Ideally, you should be aiming for 8 – 10 drinks a day, 2.5 – 3 litres per day

I was so shocked and surprised that he did not get other health problems. I got him to add more drinks throughout the day to help with his hydration and fluid levels.

We may even ask you on a scale of 1 – 10 what your energy or stress levels are, most people like to tell you a story to explain why they came up with that number on the scale.

I had a client whose energy levels were very low because of stress. She told me that she spent her nights dancing into the early hours with friends due to a very stressful job.

This was causing her to become tired due to lack of sleep and she was slowly burning out as she was burning the candle on both ends. Turned out she left her job a few months later, and is much happier now.

Take note that pain does not only come from tight muscles but it can also be emotional and physical pain as well.

All information shared is relevant even if you think it isn't, it can be the missing link to getting you out of pain.

One small change makes a difference

Ironing Lady

One client I saw a couple of years ago came to see me with a frozen shoulder and elbow pain. Upon talking to her it turned out she had a husband, and two grown children living at home and she ironed for all of them. She ironed socks, towels, pants pretty much everything and she hoovered her house every other day.

I suggested that she reduce the amount of ironing by not ironing socks, pants and towels as most of these can just be folded. In this way reducing her ironing by 25%. I also suggested that her grown children do their ironing and hoover their own thereby reducing her duties by 50%. Finally, perhaps her husband could assist with ironing some of his own items hoover every now and then. Now she was left with only 25% of the work. Guess what happened to her shoulder? The shoulder started getting better, due to her delegating work to other family members.

On Giant Shoulders

A young dad I was seeing had painful shoulders and upper back pain. One weekend he was showing me a photo of his son's birthday, in the photo the young son sat high up on the dad's shoulders holding on around his neck, he loves sitting up high he said he sits here at the weekend when we go out for the day.

...So we came up with the following plan:

He started by only allowing the child to sit on his shoulders for short periods(2 x ten minutes at a time on a Sunday over the next two weeks).

Then let him sit on the dad's shoulders once for five minutes at a time on a Sunday and over the next two weeks.

Then stop the little one from sitting on his shoulders altogether. A weight around his shoulders had now been lifted and his shoulder pain started to ease.

Jeans

Next time you're walking behind a person check out their back pockets. Men and teenage girls in particular tend to carry their wallets and mobile phones in jean back pockets. Not only is it easy to pickpocket them but have they ever thought about these items causing them lower back, lumbar and glute pain pressing against these muscles all day long.

The Morning Rave

In the city of London in old warehouses around the Shoreditch area Liverpool Street at 5.30am, high flying business men and women would gather in jeans and t–shirts and dance to high-energy rave music to -

- raise their Levels
- help them make better business decisions
- lift their mood

- feel upbeat and happy
- start their day in a positive state of mind

They would then stop, walk home, shower change into their business suits and go off to work with a spring in their step.

The first time I did this, it happened at 8.30am at a weekend marketing seminar in Coventry just after a buffet breakfast in the large hall. It had been set up with glow sticks, exercise girls on stage dancing, Conga lines forming around chairs, disco lights, beach balls, guys doing press-ups or back flips in the corner all too fast and rave music for the all-important morning rave - all this at 8.30am. I am sure the hotel guests would wonder what on earth was going on in the rooms above but the idea was to wake up to exercise, to get you up and to feel stress-free and function for the day ahead.

Most times now, I even put the radio on and have a jig around in the kitchen to an energetic song for 2 – 3 minutes and although there's no one to see me, only the cat, it does make me feel better and ready to face a new day with energy.

Try it for yourself…

EXERCISE

- Find yourself a space at home
- Find a high-energy song for 2 – 3 Minutes
- Move your body and dance
- Do you feel better?

This will also work for saying a sentence over and over for 2 minutes for motivation and upliftment.

(Reinforcing the sentence)

i.e. – I am going to mow my lawn in two hours - I am going to mow my lawn in two hours

- Say the sentence over and over again

- Find a high-energy song for 2 – 3 minutes

- Move your body

- Do you feel better?

Gratefulness

Gratefulness helps us focus our attention on the day that's been, to be grateful for things that we take for granted and those that have helped us through the day.

Take a minute or two just before eating dinner or just before going to bed to finish the day on a positive note.

People nowadays look for the next big thing they can buy, rather than what they already have.

So, we could say:

- I am grateful for the sunshine. The way it shines makes me feel great all day.

- I am very grateful to Fred for helping me with my garden this morning, it looks so much better now.

- I am grateful for the bus driver that waited for me when I ran for the bus to get me to my appointment on time.

- I am so grateful for being able to get down onto the floor and up again without any effort.

And so on ……

Making a difference

Making a difference is the little things that we do for others that make us feel great and proud that we helped.

Take a minute or two just before eating dinner or just before going to bed to finish the day on a positive note.

So, we could say:

- I am happy that I helped Mary with her shopping, we got it done a lot quicker than she would have done it alone.

- I am feeling great that I helped the blind lady cross the road, she was finding it difficult with all the traffic on the road.

- I am glad I handed the purse the staff member, that I found on the floor in the bakery, I hope the person comes back and finds it.

Deadlines

How many times have you heard?

I'll do this later…

I'll do this tomorrow…

Tomorrow never comes …….

For a deadline to work and be effective you need to:

Set a goal – Commit – Follow your plan - Take action and finish what you started.

Unless you put your foot down and say:

No, this is getting done NOW - I am mowing the lawn NOW.

- * This is getting done every morning at 7.30am. I am starting my stretching exercises at 7.30am every morning.

- * I am going to make sure that I drink 10 drinks per day, every hour or so each day.

Treat Yourself

As a great mentor once said to me "Stop being so hard on yourself".

As a rule, indeed, we are very hard on ourselves.

We keep pushing, not resting, we don't praise ourselves enough for a job or task well done.

We're fantastic with others giving advice, people pleasing going out of our way to help but what about ourselves?

Think, when did you treat yourself last?

I say this to my clients ....

What did you treat yourself to when you DID X?

What did you treat yourself to when you ACHIEVED X?

Just an acknowledgement of praise to ourselves could be:

A small treat (something you have wanted to buy), shoes, lipstick, CD, trainers or perhaps, a spa day, two hours to yourself, a walk in a beautiful park, a meal out etc.

My favourite is a bunch of lovely fresh flowers.

EXERCISE

Write on a piece of paper a goal that you would like to achieve, think of the steps below and follow suit with your own goal.

Goal - Buy a car next week

Try not to make the goal to out of reach i.e. – buying a car next week may be extreme.

It could be, I'd like to buy a car that can I afford, what can I save each month to achieve this? Work out the maths.

Think of an achievable date, so if I save £200 per month then in six months, I will have £1,200 as a deposit.

Write out six post it notes around your home in places where you will see them if you open a cupboard every day, sit in your chair, walk by, in your car, on the ceiling over your bed etc.

WRITE THIS:

I am so grateful I've saved £200 per month for six months and by x date (in six months' time), I will have £1,200 towards a deposit for my new car.

In the meantime, start looking for cars and sitting in them. It will give the goal more meaning and the goal will start becoming real.

Then when you have the money go and get your car – Enjoy the ride.

Goal – I want to lose weight by the 1st of September for my summer for my holiday

It could be I'd like to lose weight for my holiday that's on 1st September, I have X amount of time to lose X amount of weight. The longer the time to have, the better. It's not good thinking, I want to lose two stone in two weeks when I go away on 1st September.

So, think of an achievable weight to lose, in this case two stone (28 pounds). What can I lose per month over six months? 28 divided by 6 = 4.7 pounds per month that you need to lose.

Start buying better food choices and throw away all your junk food around the home. Join a slimming club and start exercising so as burn the calories quicker.

Write out six post it notes around your home in places where you will see it, if you open a cupboard every day, sit in your chair, walk by, in your car, on the ceiling over your bed etc.

I am so grateful I've lost 4.7 pounds of weight each month and by 1st September I would have lost two stones and will feel fantastic on my holiday in September.

In the meantime, go and buy a few new clothes for your holiday, the new weight size that you will achieve. This gives the goal more meaning and the reality of achieving your goal starts becoming real.

Then when you reach your new weight - Enjoy your holiday.

I've helped several clients stop smoking, lose weight, etc. with a similar strategy - as above.

Meditation

Meditation gives us space to slow down, be in the here and now, focus on our breathing and on ourselves and our feelings within our body. With Covid, Brexit, World Wars ever increasing economy, we are stressed more than ever, so meditation can help us to relax and breathe for a while.

"Go within every day and find the inner strength so that the world will not blow your candle out." Kathrine Dunham

Meditation Exercise

Sit in a quiet space on a chair or laying down on the floor or a bed, with no distractions, unplug your phone.

If you can listen to a nice relaxing piece of music this is lovely to do.

Have a look on YouTube for meditation music.

Time over 10 – 20 Minutes

- Close your Eyes
- Feel the weight of your body on the bed or chair
- Feel the weight of your legs, arms, back and head on the bed or chair
- Let them relax and just be
- Feel your hands, feet, neck, fingers, toes, face and foot
- Let them relax and just be
- Focus on your breath and your breathing, don't change it, just let it be
- If your mind starts to wander, just focus on your breath
- Try to see whether you breathing from your stomach or chest
- Relax, nice slow breathing

- Enjoy the silence, just be

- What can you hear around you? Just listen

- Keep focusing on your breath for as long as you wish

- Start to bring your focus back in the room

- Open your eyes

- Slowly shake your hands or wiggle your toes

- Slowly sit up or move around

- Drink a glass of water to ground yourself

You can find various pieces of meditation music on - **www.youtube. com** which will help you to relax

Sunshine Yellow

Yellow is the colour of happiness and joy. People with depression have long been known to wear yellow tinted glasses or wake up to a SAD lamp to lift their mood in winter months due to lack of sunshine and darker evenings.

Feel like you're missing out on the sunshine while at work? Here's a few tips to feel great about working while it's sunny.

1. Eat breakfast in the garden

2. Walk to and from the station

3. Walk from the bus stop to the office

4. Get outside on your lunch break

5. Hold a meeting outside in the park

6. Work from home - work from the garden/park

7. Instead of sitting down to watch TV when you get home, go for a walk, go for a jog, walk the dog, or wash the car

8. Eat dinner in the garden

9. Enjoy a night cap and watch the sun go down

10. Sleep with the window and blinds/curtains open for fresh air and natural light

Ways to bring yellow into your life:

1. Wear yellow clothes

2. Treat yourself to a bunch of yellow flowers

3. Buy yellow items i.e. – book, bag, bar

4. Eat yellow – Bananas, Melon

5. Paint your front door or wall yellow

Ever wondered why MacDonald's, Shell and Ikea, have yellow shop interior or big space layouts? This is because it's bright and welcoming to customers.

Managing Your Pain

Mr Ashen Face

Once in a while, I get a client who comes in to see me and their face is the colour of ash, a dark grey ill look of chronic pain. They walk clumsily, and their movements are stagnant, one shoulder higher than the other, they're not sleeping too well and the pain is draining their energy. They walk with their head down and it's a sad sight.

Sadly, people leave or stay in pain too long and decide to take action way down the line. Some want a quick fix in one or two sessions and others cut corners to pay, and finish their rehabilitation but don't stay to maintain their health, only to appear a year later standing at my door still in pain to start the process all over again.

Then I get the ever faithful that understand the power of the treatments, and stay with you for years and years.

An accident, working too long hours, early morning starts, on the go from dawn to dusk has caused this to happen, easily done.

On several occasions I've witnessed this, thinking I hope they can continue to let me treat them. I can make such a difference in their lives at the moment and get them back to health.

Then after a couple of sessions of clinical massage and a Reiki session was into the mix to rebalance and calm, then a little advice on recovery and homework to speed up the treatments the next time I see them the transformation is phenomenal. The Ash face has been replaced by a bright pinkie face, with a smile, with a glow full of life, with more movement in their body, less pain and they're sleeping like a baby.

"You Cured Me"

"You have Magic Hands"

This is what drives my motivation, this is the reason I get out of bed in the morning to help people with Ashen Faces and the many other clients I see.

The Fix Me clients and the Avoiders will learn in their sweet way that you can waste your money all you want.

CHAPTER
5

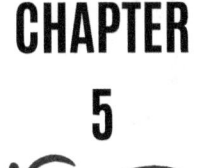

Recourses

Ball Foot Rolling

Place the ball under the sole of your naked foot while standing and roll away, not too fast you're looking for any soft or tender areas to roll over from the bridge back to the heel and under your toes. At first attempt it will probably be a little unpleasant but as time goes on the more you do it the easier it will become and the less the pain.

EXERCISE

Bend over and slowly see how far you can touch your toes. Monitor how far you can reach and how tight your hamstrings at the upper back legs feel.

Now do the Ball Rolling as above spending three minutes or so on each foot, now try again to bend over and touch your toes this time it should be a lot easier and the hamstrings in your back legs should be not so tight.

What you have done is opened up some of your artificial back line that runs from head to foot.

Ice Bottle Rolling

Fill up a plastic bottle (500ml) with water, replace the lid and freeze until solid, here you have a homemade ice pack which is great to roll on the bottom of your feet for conditions such as Plantar Fasciitis and Policeman's Heel.

Simply take it from the freezer and roll it on the bottom of your foot sole or heel area, keep the bottle moving to avoid freeze burn from the bottle.

Other uses

A hard ball or spikey ball can also be used as a mini foam roller to work on the soles of feet, hips, glutes and lumber, any tight areas that you can find while leaning against a wall and slowly working around the tight area.

A sponge or soft ball on the other hand is better for people with arthritis and gaining hand strength due to hand injuries and also great for stroke clients gaining hand grip.

Pillow Talk

Pillows have been used for comfort, to help sleep, take down any swelling and protect injured limbs while they heal.

I've even had a couple of clients bring their sleeping pillows in, to ask me if this is all right for them to be using.

Sleeping on your back

(For - lower back pain, chest injuries, and chest surgery)

Place the pillow under your knees this helps tip your pelvis, taking the pressure from your lower back and making sleeping a little more comfortable

(For - swollen feet, ankles and knees)

Place a pillow at the end of your bed and place your feet on top, your feet should now be a little higher this helps take down any swelling overnight instead of blood pooling into your feet.

Sleeping on your front

(For lower back pain)

Place a pillow under your stomach to take pressure off your lower back, this makes sleeping more comfortable.

One Pillow or Two

Sometimes a painful neck can be caused by pillows which are too high and you may find that one pillow works better but it's all about what's comfortable for you.

There are lots of different types of pillows to choose from:

soft/hard Pillows with various fillings - Memory Foam, V Pillows.

Placing Limbs on Pillows

Placing limbs on a pillow can be helpful to take down swelling, as it places the limb higher than your body and can act as a protective barrier to stop you from rolling onto it while sleeping during the night.

Stress Relievers

Stress can play a big part in our everyday lives, in some people more than others.

Here are three simple but effective exercises to help eliminate stress.

Shower it all away

Next time you jump in the shower and are stressed, let the shower water run over you, look at the water running down your body, like the water is cleaning out all your stress, onto the shower floor and down the plug hole. Imagine all your stress running down the plug hole and away with it.

Shake it all away

Clench your hands into a tight fist, imagine drawing into your fist all your stress then stretch out your hands and fingers and then for 30 seconds shake away all your stress from your hands and fingers. You could imagine the stress being a colour being shaken away - do this 3 times.

Blow it all away

Close your mouth and breath deeply in through your nose, imagine breathing in the pure, clean, fresh air, then slowly breathe out through your mouth and imagine old stagnant grey stress leaving your body, do this slowly 3 times.

Reflective Questions

What was the most valuable message you received in this chapter?

The most valuable message I received in this chapter was.

Which two things from this chapter will you try to help your pain?

1. ---

2. ---

What will you do differently from now on?

NOTES

CHAPTER
6

Making Small Changes

Making small changes can make such a big difference to your pain and posture.

Shoulder Bags

Try carrying an even balanced Rack Sack on both shoulders instead of a heavy bag on one shoulder to help and avoid shoulder pain.

Wallets and Keys

Avoid carrying your wallet, mobile phone and/or keys in the back pockets of your jeans/pants, it will help avoid lower back and glute pain.

Pickpockets will love you on the London underground if you carry on this way.

Mobile Phones

Limit your time on your mobile phone, stop looking into your lap it's doing nothing for your Clavicle neck spine muscles keep looking down.

In a train carriage of 10 people, 8 of the people had their faces on their mobile devices and 2 were reading the Metro paper. I saw this previous week, when I was on the train back from a massage job.

High Shoulder Dad's

Young Dads' stop carrying little Johnny on your shoulders, kids are heavy to carry and the weight is busting your shoulders and neck muscles.

Hip Mum's

Young Mums' stop carrying little princes/princesses on your side hip. This is why you are suffering from hip pain. They have legs and can walk.

Saggy Sofa's

Correct a Saggy Sofa and protect your back.

If you have a very soft saggy sofa chances are, it's not doing your back much good, but if you were to place a flat piece of board under the sofa cushions it makes the sofa solid, firmer and much more comfortable again.

Bed Mattresses

Bed Mattresses should be turned head to toe and flipped right over every time you change your bed this gives an even spread of wear and usage, you should also be renewed every 8 years.

Grounding

As humans in the UK, most of us lost our natural grounding ability when we started school. Aged 5 years old we put shoes on our feet as insolation and protection and almost every day from then on.

Children and adults in Africa, Asia, Aboriginal and Native America are more grounded than we will ever be as they tend to be barefoot daily in life.

Do you ever feel a little lost feel like your head is high in the sky, have headaches , are spacey or unable to be in the present, you feel out of sorts, or maybe (away with the fairies) then you may be un-grounded.

This can happen for several reasons:

- Overwhelmed

- Stress
- Chronic pain
- Tiredness
- Lack of sleep
- After having a deep body massage
- After having a healing energy session
- Sadness and depression
- Headaches

Here are three ways to come back down to earth and feel grounded:

(Being grounded can help with all the above symptoms)

- Take a cold shower as cold as you can bear is very invigorating. Then when you're dry and dressed drink a glass of plain water. Try this each morning or when needed.

- Sit or lie down and follow your breath. Breathe in through your nose and then out through your mouth, let the body lead and the mind will follow. Try this each day for 30 minutes at a time.

- Go outside barefoot and stand, lie or walk on the ground, sand, earth or grass for a time, while doing so place all your awareness into your feet. Try this for 30 minutes twice a day, it's better in the sunshine and dry weather.

- Eat something that's been grown in the ground – Potatoes, Carrots, etc.

- Drink a pint of water it's one of our natural elements (Air, Fire, Earth, Water)

Reflective Questions

What was the most valuable message you received in this chapter?

The most valuable message I received in this chapter was

....
....
....
....
....
....

Which two things from this chapter will you try to help your pain?

1 ....

2 ....

What will you do differently from now on?

....
....
....
....
....

NOTES

CHAPTER
7

Builders & Trades

Working with Builders and Trades over the years, I've learnt that a lot of your injuries and pain comes from taking shortcuts on the job that can lead to long-term pain and damage if you keep this up.

Most of the time you say, "I am too busy" or is it," I am too lazy".

Remember a physical job and exercise are two different things so this means you are not exempt from exercise or stretching.

There are a few do's and don'ts that will help you stay out of pain while working in the Trade Industry.

Do

Drink:

Make sure you drink plenty, your job is very demanding physically and requires you to drink plenty of water. You will sweat throughout your job and a lot of fluid is being lost throughout the day.

Stretch:

As much as possible over lunchtime and when you get home. The demands of reaching up high and crouching down low takes its toll on the body.

Lunchbreak:

Take a lunch break, "i am too busy" i hear you say even if you go and use the toilet, grab a drink and down a sandwich you have refuelled and downed tools for twenty minutes or so. Your job is physical you need to hydrate and refuel with good food not a tesco meal deal.

Knee Pads

So many builders suffer from knee pain, due to kneeling on them, stop it. It causes fluid under the patellar, meniscus ruptures, and cartilage scraps needed.

Hard Hat

It's there for a reason to stop knocks to your head damaging your head and neck muscles. If a brick and scaff pole hit your head, the injury can be a bit like whiplash or in some cases knock you out unconscious and stop you from knocking your head when in and under small areas.

Tidy:

Try to clean up and tidy as you go. Lots of builders trip and fall due to an untidy working area causing ankle, arm and hand injuries. If you're self-employed you cannot afford have time off work due to an injury.

Steel Toe Boots

Are sometimes not the most comfortable shoes to wear but can guard against ankle injuries and broken toes. Try wearing trainers to and from work and wearing steels on-site only, then leave them in your locker or in the van and wear them as needed.

DON'T....

Carry

A screwdriver, tools, wallet, water bottle or anything in your back pocket. This over time presses into your lower back muscles acting as a constant pressure and will result in lower back pain and your wallet getting picked.

Tool kit bag

Carrying on your shoulder. I've seen a builder on the train so packed down with his tool kit bag and spirit level he could hardly walk. Leave the tools in your van or on the job. Carrying a tool kit bag like this over time pulls down on the shoulder giving you both neck and shoulder pain.

Lean

On your knees, wear knee pads and guards, and make sure you try to stay off your knees as much as possible to stop getting fluid and bursars on the knee.

Use your back

You have probably heard the term "put your back into it" in this case do not put your back it should be "put your legs into it" what i mean by this is bend your knees when lifting and carrying items such as bricks and sandbags. Let your legs take the strain they're a lot stronger than your back. Use a wheelbarrow or trolley as much as possible.

Miss

Out on breakfast, sleep and don't take risks, be organized and stay alert.

The building game can be a dangerous place to work.

Did You Know?

The leading causes of workplace deaths in the construction industry, called the "Fatal Four" by OSHA,

Include: Falls: Electrocution, Struck-by-object and Caught-in/between roughly 36.5% of all deaths in the workplace occurred due to employees falling. This includes workers who have fallen off ladders, roofs, scaffolding, and large skyscraper construction areas.

Did You Know?

Non-fatal injuries to employees by most common accident kinds

(Non-fatal injuries reported under RIDDOR 2017/18, includes those accident kinds that account for 5% or more of the total)

Slips, Trips And Falls from Floor – 31%

Handling, Lifting And Carrying – 21%

Struck By A Moving Object – 10%

Falls From A Height – 8%

Office Workers

Working with office workers over the years I've learnt that a lot of your injuries and pain comes from not taking breaks which results from you sitting in one place for far too long. Poor posture while on the PC can also lead to long-term pain and injury over time.

Most of the time you say, "I am too busy" or is it" I am too lazy".

There are a few do's and don'ts that will help you stay out of pain while working in the office.

DO ....

Take

A break every so often, now i know time flies when you're on the pc but you need to take a break every hour, even if it's to walk around the office or put the kettle on.   Gone are the days of filing papers and walking to another desk to ask a colleague a question. We simply send them an email and file everything electronically.

Lunch

Break, get out of the office or home and go for a walk, get out in the air and feel the sunlight as it tops up your vitamin d and clears your head.

"I am too busy" - what about the colleague that takes 3 – 4 smoke breaks a day i bet they work 45 minutes less than you do a day and that's almost 4 hours a week less than you.   I bet they take their lunch break as well.

Drink

Plenty of water, keep a large bottle of water and a glass on your desk and make sure you have drunk the entire bottle before the end of the day. This will keep up your concentration and stop headaches in a stuffy office environment.

Walk

To the office from the station, remember if you're at work all day in the office this walk will be your main form of exercise for many office workers.

Tidy

Your desk as you go, lots of office staff trip and fall due to untidy working areas. They trip over cables and files other staff members would have left lying around causing ankle, arm and hand injuries.

Stretch

As often as you can. Sitting at a desk can play havoc with your back and neck. There are lots of great office desk stretches you can do to help your posture.

Look at the stretches in the neck and back in Chapter 8.

DON'T ...

Carry

A laptop or heavy paperwork on one shoulder as these pulls on the shoulder joint causing pain over time. Try to carry it in a rack sack so it's evenly balanced over both shoulders to even the weight.

Use your back

You have probably heard the term "put your back into it" in this case no not your back it should be "put your legs into it" what i mean by this is bend your knees when lifting and carrying heavy items such as, paper or stock let your legs take the strain they're a lot stronger than your back. Use a trolley as much as possible.

Sit

Too low at your pc so you're looking down at the screen, it should be at eye level. If you find it's too low you will need to raise the pc or the desk it's on to make it more comfortable.

You can get a chair bolster called a mckenzie roll for the mid back so the back isn't arching too much while you're sitting.

Miss

Out on breakfast or sleep, be organized and stay alert.

The office can be an important place for making decisions, marketing and figure work.

Did You Know?

The average office work business suffers these statistics each year:

23% - Musculoskeletal Condition such as back pain and neck pain

20 % - Minor Illness, (Coughs and Colds)

11.5% - Stress and Depression

Did You Know?

The UK economy is slowly recovering, but the country's workforce is in considerable pain.

Almost 31 million days of work were lost last year due to back, neck and muscle problems according to the Office for National Statistics (ONS).

The ONS's Labour Force Survey, which polls hundreds of thousands of people in the UK, found that musculoskeletal conditions, which include a large range of bone and joint complaints, accounted for more prolonged absences than any other ailment - 2014

Reflective Questions

What was the most valuable message you received in this chapter?

The most valuable message I received in this chapter was ....
....
....
....
....
....

Which two things from this chapter will you try to help your pain?

1 ....

2 ....

What will you do differently from now on?

....
....
....

72

....
....
....
....

NOTES

CHAPTER
8

Eating and Drinking for Health

Eating Well

Compilations of all types of foods Fruit, Veg, Protein, Carbs and Fats are great for the well-being of our bodies to help with healing.

DID YOU KNOW?

Vitamin C is vital to help with soft tissue injuries. People tend to think that oranges hold high levels of Vitamin C, when Blueberries and Strawberries are an even higher source.

A little bit of all types of foods will provide all that we need –

Protein

It doesn't all need to come from animals like meat and eggs, try these for great types of protein:

- Beans

- Lentils

- Chickpeas

- Tofu

(Anti-Inflammatory Foods)

- Pineapple - The core of the pineapple contains BROMELAIN
- Turmeric and Ginger

(Other helpful Foods)

- Beetroot – Cleans the Liver
- Pineapple – Digestion, Inflammation
- Ginger - Digestion
- Mint – Sickness & Nausea
- Nutmeg – Sedative, Seep

Tips

- Beware of sugar in cereals, jams, sauces, drinks etc
- Start looking at labels on foods and packets- Be wise in getting food.
- Watch out for hidden fats and salt.

How Much Water?

I am always asking my clients "How much water do you drink daily?"

I was shocked when a client told me he averages around 3 cups of tea a day and that's it. He was quite unaware of the consequences to his health and just took the look of shock on my face on the chin.

Water helps us in many ways. Many people take medication and the water makes sure these medications are distributed around the body to all the right parts. Water takes vital nutrients around the body. Not only is water great for your skin, nails, hair and bright eyes but also helps with inflammation and pain.

Ideally, we should be drinking around 8 – 10 drinks per day be it water, tea and juices etc.

From 7.00am to 2.00pm – 4 - 5 Drinks

From 3.00pm to 10.00pm – 4 - 5 Drinks

Try to mix your drinks not just tea, tea, tea. Little and often is a great way to think.

- Remember if you feel thirsty or feel the need to drink, you're already starting to dehydrate.

A great way to get a few more glasses in is to:

- As you get up out of bed and pop to the bathroom make a detour to the kitchen and grab a quick pint of water.
- Add a drink with your meals Breakfast, Lunch and Dinner.
- Drink on tea breaks and lunch breaks.
- Drink before exercising or doing your stretches
- Google Apps on your phone has water apps that you can download which rings each hour reminding you to drink.

If you find water boring, jazz it up with:

- a slice of Cucumber, Lime, Lemon, Mint, Fruit etc

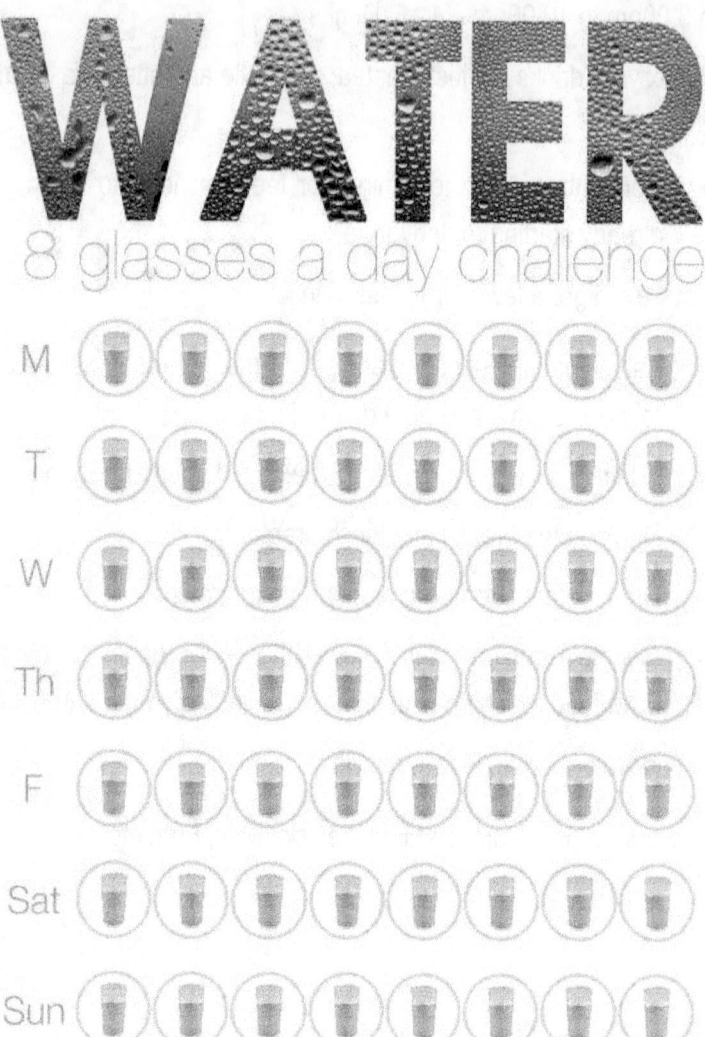

Try this for a week and see and feel the difference

Vitamins, Minerals and Arnica

Most of our diets, if you're eating well should contain most of the vitamins and minerals needed for our body's health and well-being.

Here is a list of vitamins and minerals that will help with pain and injuries:

- Vitamin B – Lacking Energy

- Vitamin D – Bone, Wellbeing

- Calcium – Bone Healing, Teeth, Strength

- Vitamin C – Tissue and Skin Healing, Immune System

- Zinc – Tissue and Skin Healing

A good all-round strong vitamin and mineral supplement can be taken while the pain is at its worst or while the body is healing.

Sugar

(The devil in the white dress) cut sugar and you'll be laughing. It's used so much and holds us back so much, progress that can be made with our health is hindered by SUGAR. It makes our bodies vulnerable to disease and obesity.

High Blood Pressure, Heart, Diabetes, Teeth, Weight, Inflammation etc.

Arnica

Witch Hazel was what we used as kids, a colourless smelling liquid that we dapped on bumps and scraps – nowadays it's Arnica.

Arnica is a flower homoeopathy helping with soft tissue healing, bruising and shock after surgery, accidents and injuries. It can be used before or after the occasion and is available from a health food store or chemist usually sold as - 30cc tablets or as a cream rub on.

How much sleep do we need?

How much sleep?

How much sleep should we be having every night? Most of us need an average of 7 – 9 hours, however, we may lose hours due to illness, celebrations, raves and plane flights where sleep sometimes goes out the window.

We recover, grow and repair while we sleep and is vital to our well–being

Power Naps

A lot of business people, school children and people throughout the world take power naps in the afternoon to rest, recharge and destress. It is also great for decision making.

DID YOU KNOW?

We are 1cm taller in the morning than in the evening. This is due to the cartilage in our knees and spine compressing as we walk around, and then it goes back to normal after rest or when we sleep.

We basically spend our 24 Hours as follows:

- 8 x Hours – Living

- 8 x Hours – Sleeping

- 8 x Hours – Working

We sleep better if our bedrooms are –

- Cool

- Dark

- Fresh air

- Comfortable Mattress

- No Television

- No Mobile Phones

DID YOU KNOW?

We are supposed to change our bed mattress every 8 years so that it doesn't start affecting our backs – When did you change your mattress last?

Is smoking costing you your health

Cigarette smoking causes premature death: Life expectancy for smokers is at least 10 years shorter than for non-smokers.

How Smoking Affects Healing:

Nicotine is a vasoconstrictor that reduces nutritional blood flow to the skin, resulting in tissue and impaired healing of injured tissue.

Smoking and wound healing:

Cigarette smoke is filled with harmful chemicals Smoking increases the chance that your bones and tissue may not heal well, may become infected, or that you may have **MORE PAIN THAN YOU DID BEFORE.**

Why people Smoke – I've heard

I am Stressed)
I am Bored
It's now a Habit
I don't know why It looks good
I am in Pain

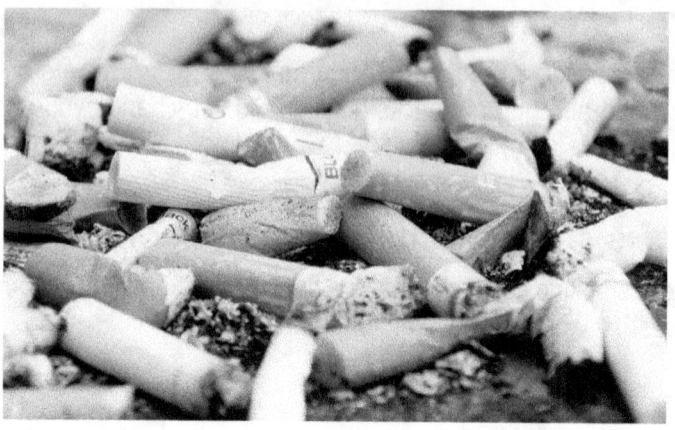

CUTTING DOWN

I've helped a few clients cut their smoking this way -

Take note that after the age of 40, it's harder to reverse the damage, so stop now before it's too late

EXERCISE

1. Break each cigarette in half and throw the top half away, this way you're saving and smoking half the amount. Use half the cigarette as if it was a whole one.

2. So, you're now down to an average of 10 x per day then cut back 1 – 2 – 3 from here

3. Look for the reasons why you're smoking i.e. habit, stress, or boredom and address them. Take up a new hobby. Start changing things for the better.

4. Get your partner to stop with you, it's hard if one of you is still smoking heavily.

5. So, before you think that maybe massage and exercise aren't working think again, maybe it's you, your smoking and healing

process that's stopping things.

6. Treat and praise yourself if you manage to cut down and stop, it's quite big thing to do.

Your weight can hinder your health

Knees

A lot of my clients suffer from knee problems and find that after losing some weight their knee pain and inflammation is a lot better – a miracle.

Cutting down on cheese, bread, potatoes, pastries and cakes makes a huge difference in the size of your legs and the weight on your knees.

Lower Back Pain

I knew a work colleague that was having a lot of lower back pain due to her bust size and had to have a bust reduction to help with her back pain.

On The Massage Treatment

Occasionally I'll get a twenty plus stone client on my table and they come for pain management. There is still plenty that I can do. Yes, they are harder to work on and move around but really their weight is an issue and they tend to know this.

During the Covid lockdown, I lost 3 Stone (20 Kilos). Years of 10k runs over weekends and the odd snack was starting to take its toll on my knees.

I've also had clients lose over a stone or so in weight just by taking simple actions such as increasing water and cutting back on sugar etc.

Reflective Questions

What was the most valuable message you received in this chapter?

The most valuable message I received in this chapter was

....
....
....
....
....
....
....

Which two things from this chapter will you try to help your pain?

1 ....

2 ....

What will you do differently from now on?

....
....
....
....
....

Notes

CHAPTER
9

Neck Pain

Think Tank

While you have a few minutes it's a good idea to ask yourself a couple of Questions:

Do I know why I've got neck pain?

It could be caused by an accident, working too long, carrying a heavy bag on the shoulder, stress, not stretching, not exercising, ironing too much, pillows too high, carrying children on shoulders, tilting neck to one side while talking on the phone, sleeping under a cold window etc.

When the Neck Pain started what you were doing at the time?

1 week ago - from a car crash or accident.

10 years ago, from working too long hours on a PC.

What can I start doing or putting in place to stop my neck pain?

- Start an exercise and stretching my neck 3 times a week and going for a walk.

- Stop ironing everything, start getting other family members to do their own ironing.

- Stop carrying your heavy bag on one shoulder and buy a rack sack to balance the weight.

Has my neck pain got worse over time? Is my range of rotation (turn) not as good as it was? Why is this?

Due to life changes, lack of exercise – ask yourself why, what changed.

It only takes two weeks to stop the habit of exercise and stretching due to getting a cold, going on holiday and getting out of your routine, and fitness starts to decrease.

Out Of 1 – 10 - How do you feel about your neck pain?

Bad - 1 2 3 4 5 6 7 8 9 10 - Good

I need to change to help my neck pain!

Change your Habits – We know what we should be doing to help ourselves we just need a guide and helping hand, follow this guide for the quickest way out of neck pain

- Stop smoking so much

- You need more exercise

- You need to stretch more

- You need more water intake

- You need to relax more

- You need more sleep

- You need to work less or smarter

Things that are not helping my neck pain at the moment

1. I am still sleeping with 2 pillows

2. I am carrying my heavy bag to work every day

3. I am letting my grandchildren sit on my shoulders

4. I am not doing my neck stretching exercises twice a day as needed

5. I am spending far too long on the PC without taking breaks

6. I am not putting heat around my neck everyday

Things I can do to help my neck pain

1. I have moved down to 1 pillow

2. I am carrying a lighter bag and have changed to a rack sack

3. I've stopped my grandchildren sitting on my shoulders now

4. I am doing my neck stretches twice a day

5. I am taking breaks and walking around for 10 minutes at work

6. I am putting heat around my neck every day to help

Neck Pain Tips

- The worst thing to do is go to bed and lay down all day.

- Keep mobile by taking short walks but also take a few rest breaks and don't sit for too long.

- Try to be as natural as possible by turning your neck when you need to, not the whole body.

- Try stretching a few times a day preferably morning and evening.

- Do not sit all day at the computer or watching television, the neck stays in one position too long.

- Neck pain is worse with stiffness in the morning when getting up as you will have been laying still sleeping for 8 hours, also early evening as you start getting tired.

- Keep lifting to a minimum until you feel a little better so, no gym, lifting shopping or small children,

- Get 8 hours sleep the body heals while sleeping – 10pm to 7am is great.

- Take your time, don't rush, slow down it may take longer to move, dress and shower and move around.

- Think of joining a Fitness class or Yoga group when you're feeling better and keep it going.

- Stretching and gentle movement is the key to your recovery.

Life Style Changes

- Take your time, don't rush, slow down it may take longer to move, dress and shower and move around.

- Try using just 1 pillow instead of 2 while sleeping to place your neck in a comfortable position for sleeping.

- Take time to relax with some meditation or deep breathing, neck pain can be stressful.

- Try to limit appointments, social events and making important decisions until you feel better.

- If you have to take a pain killer, Paracetamol is the kindest to your body while others will cause side effects. After a couple of days, you should find you need less or none at all.

Things to Stop

- Carrying your laptop bag or handbag on one shoulder, try getting a rucksack on both shoulders.

- Carrying children high on your shoulders, it's still a weight.

- Sitting at the computer or watching television for a long time.

- Try changing pillows from 2 to 1.

- Ironing everything for all the family, older children can do their own.

- Slouching on a saggy old chair or sofa in the evening, think about your posture.

Remember -

- Nothing will get better and improve unless you are willing to change and put the work into it. Do your exercise and stretches and take advice from the tips given, it's all here to help you.

- Do the stretches to your best ability and hold for a full minute, not just 15 seconds. Each exercise or stretch needs to be done 3 times , each leg/side, this all should take 20 minutes twice a day.

  One of my client's pain didn't get better until I physically did the exercises with her, she wasn't stretching far enough or long enough and was not using heat. A few days later she was fine, moving better and back to work.

- Start slowly and start adding new changes to your life as you go along, remember why you got your neck pain in the beginning, change your habits and get rid of the pain for good.

- Food and water are your friend, eat and drink the right quality and quantity.

- Sleep is vital, don't go to bed in the early hours of the morning and try to skip through on 6 hours of sleep.

- If you're doing things right you should start seeing a difference in a few days.

- If you go off track, just get back to this as soon as possible. If it's not working be honest with yourself - are you doing the best you can? Can you change to do better, a habit, stretch, stop smoking, sleep more, using heat e.t.c?

Stretches for - Neck Pain

(Take 20 minutes to do these)

- Make sure to do these neck stretches 2 times a day, repeat 2/3 times on each side.

- Try heating the neck first with a heat pack, hot water bottle or wheat bag before doing these stretches. After this the neck will move better with less pain.

1. NECK ROTATIONS

Slowly turn your head to the left holding for 1 minute, then turn right holding for 1 minute, use 2 fingers on the jawline to push your neck around – Repeat.

Doing this stretches your neck muscles by rotating from left to right.

2. NOSE TO NIPPLE

Slowly try to put your nose on your left nipple, hold for 1 minute then bring the nose to the right nipple and hold for 1 minute, press down on your head for more of a stretch if needed – Repeat.

Doing this stretches your upper shoulders and neck muscles

3. LATERAL FEX

Tilt left neck to the left shoulder and pull the head down with your left hand and hold for 1 minute REPEAT on the right side – Repeat.

Doing this, stretches the sides of your neck.

4. CHIN TO CHEST

Touch your chin on your upper chest place a hand on top of your head for more of a stretch, hold for 1 minute - Repeat.

Doing this stretches down the back of the neck, shoulders and spine.

Remember to Breathe

1 – Neck Rotations

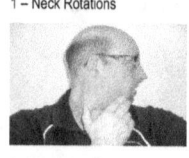

2 – Nose To Nipple

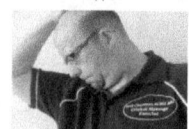

3 - Lateral Flex

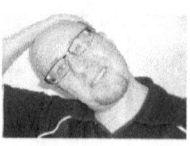

4 - chin to

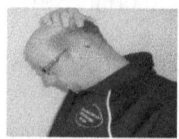

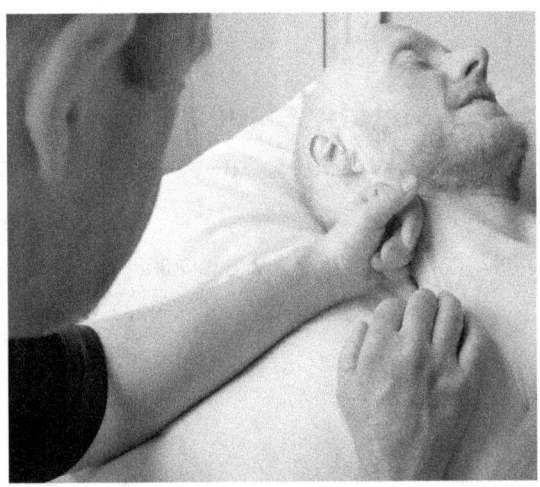

Jack Chapman ACMT

Photo by – Johnny-Dean Pearce

Questions to think about

- What can I do now to start making changes?

- What do I need to buy to start helping myself?

- What can I get ready to follow this neck plan?

- Can I start making time for myself?

- Can I think about my neck pain and how it came about?

- How far can I move my neck? how long has it been like this?

- Do I want to be free from pain in my neck?

- Am I ready and in a good place to start this neck pain plan?

NOTES

Reflective Questions

What was the most valuable message you received in this chapter?

The most valuable message I received in this chapter was

....
....
....
....
....
....
....

Which two things from this chapter will you try to help your pain?

1. ....

2. ....

What will you do differently from now on?

....
....
....
....
....

CHAPTER
10

Leg and Knee Pain

- **LEG EXTENSIONS**

  This is great for building strength in the legs to protect the knee. Sit on a chair and extend your left leg like doing a seated kick, hold the leg in this parallel position for five seconds then lower back down, do 20, reps then change to the right leg.

- **QUAD STRETCH**

  Stand holding on to a wall for balance, with your left hand grab your left ankle and pull the leg up behind you, so the leg is bent almost in half and hold. Feel the stretch on the front quad (thigh muscle) hold for 1 minute, then do this 3 times then repeat on the right leg.

- **HIP SWINGS**

  Stand holding on to a wall for balance, with your left leg swing the left leg back and forward or out to the side as well giving movement into the hip and lower back, do 20 times, then repeat on the right leg

- **SQUATS**

  The all-around leg builder, you should feel this in most of your leg and glute muscles. Stand with feet parallel to the floor, and bend your knees, your knees should just be over your feet, remember to keep your back straight, do 2 x 20 with a minute rest.

- Remember to breathe.

- KNEE PAIN: If you make yourself lighter in body weight and your legs stronger,your thighs, hamstrings and your knees will be less achy and painful overall.

Leg Extension	Quad Stretch	Hip Swing
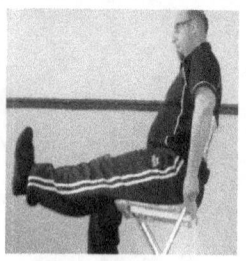	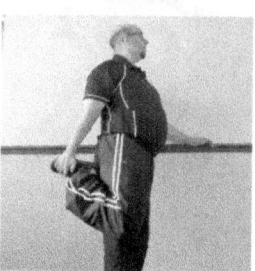	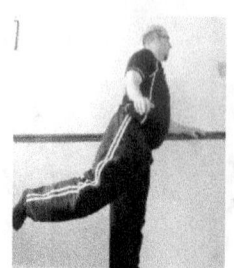

squats

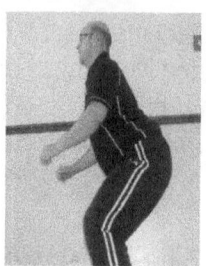

Shoulder Pain

- **PENDULUM SWINGS**

   Great one for frozen shoulder and lack of shoulder movement. Bend over a table or chair and let the arm and hand hang loose; slowly start swinging the right arm side to side and back and forward just like a pendulum clock movement, do this for 3 – 5 minutes on the affected shoulder to gain back direction.

- **FINGER WALKING**

   Again great one for lack of shoulder movement. Stand facing a wall, place your hand on the wall and start walking your fingers up the wall, rest for a few seconds DO NOT MOVE YOUR HAND FROM THE WALL, then go up higher again until you can go no higher, you may have to step into the wall to go higher, then slowly lower by sliding your arm and hands down the wall and repeat several times.

- **SIDE LATERAL RAISES**

  In a standing position try raising your left arm with the palm facing down up towards your head and reach upwards towards the ceiling with the arm straight at the elbow, do this serveral times on the affected side.

- **DOORWAY STRETCH**

  Great for computer workers and people with rounded shoulders. Stand in between a doorway, place both your inner forearms on the doorway frame, place one leg forward bent at the knee through the doorway, push through the doorway as you push feel the stretch across your front chest and shoulder muscles and hold for 1 minute.

  - Remember to breathe

  - Try NOT to carry a bag on the affected shoulder or do any ironing
    - etc

Pengulum Swings   Finger Walking   Side Lateral Raises

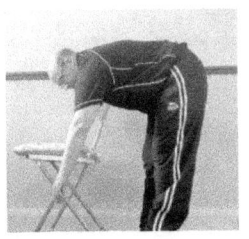 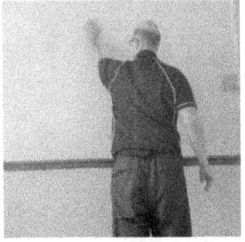 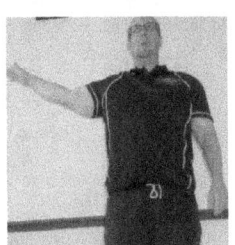

Doorway Stretch

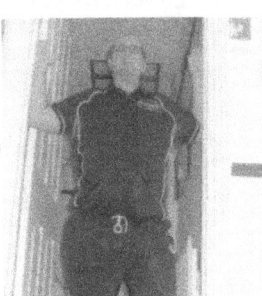

Elbow Pain & Grip Pain

Elbow and grip pain can be brought on by not only playing tennis and golf.

It can be brought on by overusing your arms and hands (RSI) with tasks such as

Hoovering, ironing, computer work, painting, using tools, and repetitive movements etc.

- This Injury is usually helped with ICE over the elbow area.

- **Tennis Elbow**

  For pain on the lateral (outside) of the elbow place the fingers down and stretch the wrist down (Tennis Elbow).

  The arm has to be straight at the elbow for it to work, you can use the other hand to assist the stretch for more pressure, hold for 1 minute and repeat several times.

- **Golfers Elbow**

  For pain on the medial inside of the elbow place the fingers up and stretch the wrist upwards (Golfers Elbow).

  The arm has to be straight at the elbow for it to work, you can use the other hand to assist the stretch for more pressure, hold for 1 minute and repeat several times.

- **Grip Pain**

  Grip Pain is usually caused by (RSI) many repeated movements and gripping actions such as using tools, it can be helped by stretching out the hands, wrists, fingers and loosening the tight muscles in the forearm.

Golfers elbow   Tennis Elbow   Grip Pain

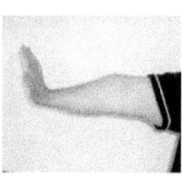
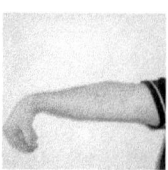
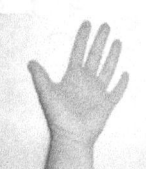

Ankle Pain & Plantar Fasciitis

Ankle and Planter pain (foot sole/heel) can be due to a number of reasons.

They include ,drop foot, fall, rolled ankle or twisted ankle, Achilles Tendon injury standing or walking on hard floors for a long time.

*ICE - is usually used with the ankle and foot sole & heel pain to help swelling and bruising. Plantar Fasciitis can also feel red, needle stabbing in the heel and a burning like sensation. Elevating the legs on a pillow or stool can also help with swelling around the ankles.

- **Step Calf Raises**

  Stand on a step or the bottom (NOT TOP) step of a staircase, stand on the edge of the step with your toes, but enough that you wouldn't slip off.

  Slowly raise up on your toes as high as you can and hold for a second or so then raise back to parallel and then let your heels lower to get the stretch up your ankle and calf muscles – 3 times 30 within a 1-minute rest in-between.

- **Ankle Flex**

  Sit on a chair and lift your leg like doing a seated kick, place an exercise band or cord under the sole of your foot, holding on to the band or cord with both hands. Pull the foot back and hold for a few seconds, then reverse this action and point the toes forward and hold for a few seconds, repeat this several times

- **Plantar Fasciitis & Heel Pain**

  Tip: Freeze a 500ml bottle of water and roll the foot sole and heel over the bottle to cool and work the area. You can also use a spiky massage ball then do calf raises to stretch the foot sole, try to rest by staying off your feet.

Step Calf Raises   Ankle Flex   Plantar Fasciitis

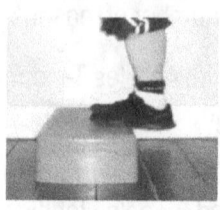 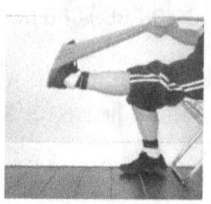 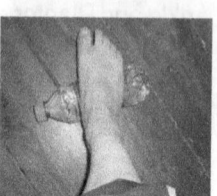

Back Pain

Think Tank

While you have a few minutes it's a good idea to ask yourself a couple of questions:

Do I know why I've got lower back pain?

- An accident or an injury ?
- Working too long sitting at a PC?
- Not stretching or exercising?
- Carrying a wallet in my back trouser pocket?
- Sitting on a saggy sofa watching too much evening television?

When the lower back pain started what you were doing at the time?

- 1 week ago - from a car crash, accident or gardening
- 5 years ago, from lack of Exercise
- 10 years ago, from working too long hours on a PC

What can I start doing or putting in place to stop my lower back pain?

- Start exercise and stretching my back 3 times a week and start going for a walk.

- Stop working on the PC for long hours without taking tea breaks and lunch breaks.

- Stop carrying keys, phone and wallet in back pockets, this pushes on the back muscles.

Out Of 1 – 10 - How do you feel about your back pain?

Bad - 1 2 3 4 5 6 7 8 9 10 – Good

I need to change to help my back pain!

Change your habits – We know what we should be doing to help ourselves we just need a guide and helping hand, follow this guide for the quickest way out of lower back pain.

- Stop smoking so much, quit if you can

- You need to change your bad habits

- You need more exercise

- You need to stretch more

- You need more water intake

- You need to relax and sleep more

- You need to work less or smarter

Things that are not helping my lower back pain at the moment

1. I am tired when I get home from work so I chill out all evening on our saggy old sofa watching television or reading, I guess I am not moving enough.

2. I am carrying my wallet and keys in my back trouser pocket and it's pushing on my glute muscles which is not helping my back.

3. I am sitting long hours on my PC without any breaks, I guess that's why I am stiff.

4. I am not doing my lower back stretching twice a day that is why I am not better

5. I am not doing any other form of exercise because my job is physical and I think this is enough.

6. I am not icing and heating my lower back as needed every day to help my swelling or circulation.

7. I not going to bed until 1am and I am only just getting 6 hours sleep, I hear sleep is one thing needed for recovery.

Things that are helping my lower back pain

1. I try to sit upright with my lower back pain and move around every few minutes.

2. I've stopped carrying my wallet and keys in my back trouser pocket.

3. I am now taking breaks and not sitting for too long on my PC.

4. I am stretching my lower back twice every day.

5. I've stopped smoking and I am eating clean foods and drinking more water.

6. I am walking in my local park every evening getting some movement in my lower back.

7. I am icing and heating my lower back.

8. I am in bed by 10pm to get my full 8 hours sleep.

Back Pain Tips

- Take your time, don't rush, slow down it may take longer to move, dress and shower and walk around.

- Try placing a pillow or foam roller under your knees while sleeping to tip your pelvis and place you in a comfortable position for sleeping.

- Take time to relax with some meditation or deep breathing, back pain can be stressful.

- Try to limit appointments, social events and making important decisions until you feel better.

- If you have to take a pain killer, Paracetamol is the kindest to your body, others will cause side effects. After a couple of days, you should find you need less or none at all.

- With spasms, try not to panic, take your time, and go slow it feels terrible and very painful and even frightening, the key is to relax and breathe and ice the area for 15 minutes at a time with a bag of frozen peas in a plastic bag. Do this for 2 days   DO NOT use heat at this time. The ice should calm and stop the spasms.

- Make sure you keep drinking water; the more you sweat the more you need to drink.

- Do not go to bed and lay there all, day this is the worst thing to do, you need to move.

- Find ways of dressing easier for a few days, putting on joggers or slip-on shoes.

- Try to dress, shower and get out for a short walk it will make you feel better.

- Try moving your lower back as naturally as possible, don't be stiff and ridged.

- Make sure you do your stretches - this is the key to recovery.

- Make changes and create new habits now, I am sure this is something you will never want to go through again in a hurry.

- Book in with us for a FREE 30 minute lower back consultation Call - 07860 227774

Remember

- Nothing will get better and improve unless you are willing to change and put the work in to it. Do your exercises and stretches and take advice from the tips given, it's all here to help you.

- Do the stretches to your best ability and hold for a full 1 minute, not just 15 seconds. Each exercise/stretch needs to be done 3 times , on each leg/side, this all should take 20 minutes twice a day.

- Start slowly and start adding new changes to your life as you go along, remember why you got your back pain in the beginning, change your habits and get rid of the pain for good.

- If you're doing everything well, you should start to see a difference in a few days to a week.

- Food and water are your friends, eat and drink good quality and enough.

- Sleep is vital, don't go to bed in the early hours of the morning.

- Try to sleep at least 6 hours because sleep is vital for recovery and repair.

- If you go off track, just get back to this as soon as possible. It's not the end of the world, just start again. If it's not working be honest, are you doing the best you can? Can you change to do better, a habit, smoking, sleep more, walking etc.?

Things to Stop

- Carrying your wallet, mobile or keys in the back trouser pocket.

- Sitting on the computer or watching television for too long.

- Smoking – this will delay your healing and increase your pain.

- Slouching on a saggy old chair or sofa in the evening.

- Lifting and carrying without thinking about your body, bend your knees, and let your legs take the strain not your back.

Lower Back Stretches

(15 Minutes)

- You must do these lower back stretches 2 times a day – Both AM and PM.

- Try doing these after heating or icing it will be less painful and the back will move better, your back will feel stiff more in the morning as you've been in bed for 8 hours and in the early evening as you're starting to get tired.

- If getting on the floor is too much, try stretching on your bed, hold each position for 1 minute, change legs and repeat several times on each side, take your time, relax don't rush or skip these stretches they are part key to your recovery.

1. KNEE TO CHEST

Lay on the floor or bed and bring your left knee to your chest, relax and hold it here for 1 minute and repeat on the right leg, repeat again on each side.

2. SPINAL TWIST

Lay on the floor, bring your left foot across your right knee and place on the floor, with your right hand on your left knee slowly pull your knee across towards the floor on your right side the more you pull the more you stretch the lower back and glutes. You can put your left arm out to the side and turn your head to look to the right to deepen the stretch - Hold for 1 minute and repeat on the right side.

3. CHILDS POSE

Get onto your knees on the floor or on the bed and sit back onto your lower legs and heels. Stretch out your arms out in front of you so you are low on the floor or bed, relax and hold for 1 minute – Repeat several times.

4. CAT AND COW STETCH

Get onto your knees on the floor or bed and arch your back up like a cat bringing your chin to your chest tuck in your neck – hold for 30 seconds then reverse this position by sticking your bottom out behind you and bringing your head up - look up to the ceiling, relax and hold for 30 seconds – repeat doing this several times.

Knee to Chest Spinal Twist Child's Pose

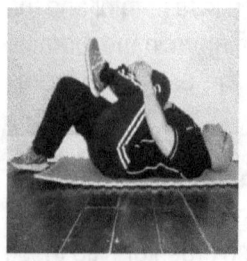 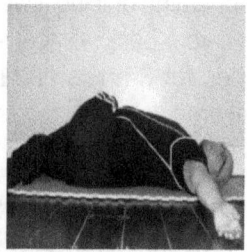 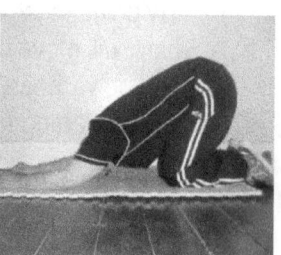

Cat & Cow

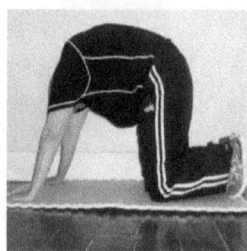

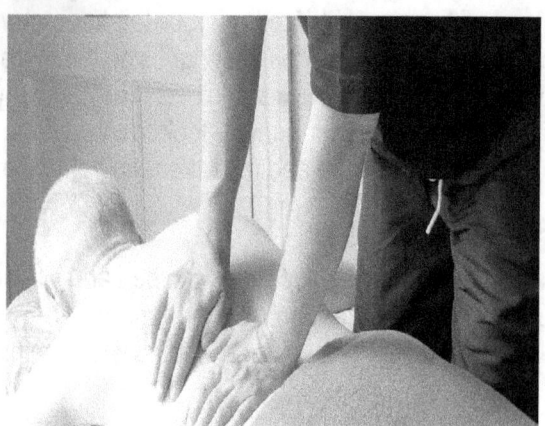

Jack Chapman ACMT

Photo by – Johnny- Dean Pearce

Questions

- What can I do now to start making changes?
- What do I need to buy to start helping myself?
- What can I get ready to follow this lower back plan?
- Can I start making time for myself?
- Can I think about my lower back pain and how it came about?
- Do I want to be free from pain in my lower back?
- Am I ready and in a good place to start this lower back pain plan?

Reflective Questions

What was the most valuable message you received in this chapter?

The most valuable message I received in this chapter was

....
....
....

Which two things from this chapter will you try to help your pain?

1. ....

2. ....

What will you do differently from now on?

....
....
....
....

NOTES

The Most Important Part

Consistency is the key word here, little and often is sometimes the only way forward. Learn the hard way or the easy way to get out of pain.

(Keep On, Keep On as one of my great massage trainers would say and yes she was right!)

Each day, it may seem like an endless task to get up early to stretch, do your exercises, ice or heat an area. To get food and liquids ready, feeding your body with the best nutrition to help it heal, put new plans and habits in place, go for a walk after work when all you want to do is crash and watch television or go to bed early when the late-night football is on.

Good habits, discipline and consistency are supposed to be your friends.

Laziness, not planning ahead are your enemies.

Back in 2020 I lost just over 3 stone; I took it to the extreme like I do when I really want something. My goal was to look good, be healthy and to see my abdominal muscles that I hadn't seen for years, since my competitive bodybuilding days.

Yes, it was hard at first a but the results and scales kept me motivated and with that end goal in mind, this should be the same for you, feeling healthier, painless and striving to be better. We aren't getting any younger and our health is should be top priority.

Putting it all together

So, by now you can see the pattern beginning to emerge with pain and injuries. It isn't just a case of doing a couple of stretches a few times a week. That will help but will not be the overall answer. These are the people that will never heal or take a while to heal or will eventually to do more to help themselves.

It's a combination of having a plan in place, getting together anything, you need i.e., hot cold packs, exercise band, joining classes gym, buying a diary etc. Have someone to keep you accountable for doing these next few steps, don't stop just keep on doing all these things, this may be a therapist or a coach., Ask yourself questions about why or how the pain happened and keep a pain diary of how you're progressing. Some form of exercise, stretching, strength work if needed, using heat and ice if needed, eating, and drinking enough and the suitable types of foods, getting enough rest and sleep, making sure you are not stressed, getting sunshine and fresh air, taking time for you and slowly it will start coming together. Changing the habits within your work, family life and overall lifestyle for the better.

We all know that things happen, you go to a party and have a couple of drinks, go to bed late and wake up late the next day. In the winter, it's a cold Monday morning you don't feel like getting up at 6 am to do that early morning walk that was a joy this time around in the summer. That's life, but it doesn't mean you failed, and it's not the end of the world, if anything you've relaxed and taken time out for you. As long as it's within moderation and doesn't become a new habit, just get back up, get back on the rolling wagon, and start again with your plan and keep going until you get the results you need.

Spend a bit of time being honest and truthful with yourself. Ask yourself a few home truths about what can you do to help yourself and progress forward without reverting backwards. It may help to have a light and shadow chart listing 6 things to start doing i.e., (Light)" I plan to do my stretching at 7am each morning and set my alarm clock." (Shadow) "I won't get better without doing my stretching at 7am each morning and setting my alarm clock to get me up." (Light) "I plan to drink a pint of water each morning on rising to hydrate myself." (Shadow) "If I don't drink enough water each day my pain will stay around for longer. "Maybe write it down then say it out loud to yourself, it will help cement the healing plan.

Most people I talk to know the basics and know that they should be doing more to help themselves. The plan is right within this book, and the rest is up to you with a loving kick up the jacksie.

Reflective Questions

What was the most valuable message you received in this chapter?

The most valuable message I received in this chapter was ......

....
....
....
....
....
....

Which two things from this chapter will you try to help your pain?

1. ....
....

2. ....
....

What will you do differently from now on?

....
....
....
....

Notes

About the Author

Jack Chapman lives and works in South East London and Kent UK.

He has influenced and helped hundreds of people over the years running his own business as an Advanced Clinical Massage Therapist, Stroke Rehabilitation Trainer, Reiki Healer and Exercise Instructor in his local area.

Having a 20 year background before in Public Customer Services, Diplomatic Security, and the Art and Fitness Industry, Jack loves helping people solve their problems, finding solutions and helping to change their lives for the better.

He has said to one client that asked him "Will you give up on me like the last Physio Trainer? -His reply was "You'll give up long before I ever give up on you."

One lady said, "you'll be shocked at my lack of movement and saggy neck skin." Jack's reply was "After seeing a human dissection autopsy in a London hospital for massage training, working in Diplomatic Security and the Art Industry not a lot shocks me nowadays."

His work and training have taken him all over the UK and Europe, finding and discovering new ideas, methods and ways to help himself help others with chronic pain conditions, which he continues with today.

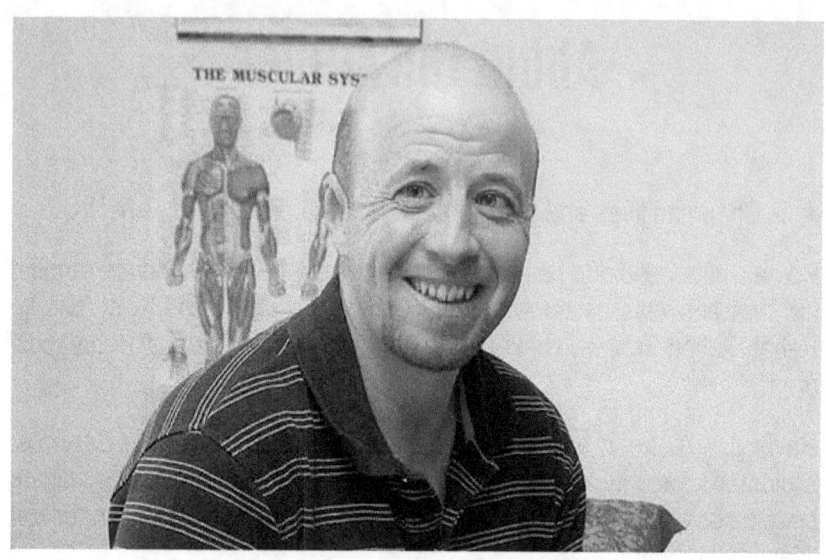

A personal message from Jack

I hope this book has inspired you and you will use it as a tool.The words, personal stories, suggestions, helpful tips and exercises in this book will help you live a healthy and fulfilled life which is free of pain as much as possible.

Tears flowed a few times while writing this book, with lots of thoughts from the past. Old clients that I'd started with and helped in Care Homes that are no longer with us and the fantastic progress that had been made by clients that have tried and successfully helped themselves get better both with rehabilitation and finally out of pain, and my thoughts and views and life in general.

Going alone into the self-employment business from a different industry can be a tough call. I would tell anyone trying to do so on their own to build a strong network around them, seek out the best training advice you can afford and a good marketing mentor that has the skills you need, they are worth their weight in gold as it can make or break your business.

If you love your job, it's something that you can get great pleasure from and are handsomely rewarded. During the time of writing this book Covid has hit the world and it is a very trying time for us all, we all have a story to tell but keep moving forward. I am still running my full-time Advanced Clinical Massage Practice, Stroke Rehabilitation Training and Exercise Sessions within my local area.

If you have enjoyed this book feel free to spread the word to your family, friends and colleagues so they too can be helped with their pain and gain knowledge into helping themselves to live a healthy lifestyle.

I hope this book has inspired you and you will use it as a tool.Jack x

Contact

Contact me for help and advice – Jack Chapman

Facebook

Jack Chapman ACMT Pain & Injury Clinic – Welling, Kent

E Mail

therapy.heaven@yahoo.co.uk

Website

www.jackchapman.info

End